DETOX YOUR HOME

DETOX YOUR HOME

A Guide to Removing
Toxins from Your Life
and Bringing Health
into Your Home

CHRISTINE DIMMICK

ROWMAN & LITTLEFIELD
Lanham • Boulder • New York • London

Published by Rowman & Littlefield
A wholly owned subsidary of The Rowman & Littlefield Publishing Group, Inc.
4501 Forbes Boulevard, Suite 200, Lanham, Maryland 20706
www.rowman.com

Unit A, Whitacre Mews, 26-34 Stannary Street, London SE11 4AB

British Library Cataloguing in Publication Information Available

Library of Congress Cataloging-in-Publication Data
Names: Dimmick, Christine, author.
Title: Detox your home : a guide to removing toxins from your life and
   bringing health into your home / Christine Dimmick.
Description: Lanham : Rowman & Littlefield, [2018] | Includes bibliographical
   references and index.
Identifiers: LCCN 2018006026 (print) | LCCN 2018006664 (ebook) | ISBN
   9781442277212 (electronic) | ISBN 9781442277205 (cloth : alk. paper)
Subjects: LCSH: Toxins—Physiological effect. | Detoxification (Health)
Classification: LCC RA1250 (ebook) | LCC RA1250 .D56 2018 (print) | DDC
   615.9/5—dc23
LC record available at https://lccn.loc.gov/2018006026

∞™ The paper used in this publication meets the minimum requirements of
American National Standard for Information Sciences—Permanence of Paper
for Printed Library Materials, ANSI/NISO Z39.48-1992.

Printed in the United States of America

DEDICATION

This book is dedicated to all those who work tirelessly to protect our planet and our health, who continuously go on, without acknowledgment, support, or personal gain—but only for the reason it is the right thing to do.

> On all farms, farmers would undertake to know responsibly where they are and to "consult the genius of the place." They would ask what nature would be doing there if no one were farming there. They would ask what nature would permit them to do there, and what they could do there with the least harm to the place and to their natural and human neighbors. And they would ask what nature would help them to do there. And after each asking, knowing that nature will respond, they would attend carefully to her response. The use of the place would necessarily change, and the response of the place to that use would necessarily change the user. The conversation itself would thus assume a kind of creaturely life, binding the place and its inhabitants together, changing and growing to no end, no final accomplishment, that can be conceived or foreseen.

> Berry, Wendell. *Bringing It to the Table*, 2009. Part 1, Farming, page 8.

CONTENTS

ACKNOWLEDGMENTS

THIS BOOK would not exist if not for Shannon Drenik and Patricia Helding. Thank you Shannon for putting me on the path and your endless support and encouragement. Thank you Pat for seeing a book, leading me to Sharon, and your unwavering support of my work. You are both angels on earth, and I am blessed to know you. I thank you Sharon Bowers for believing in this with all your heart—because you believed this information needed to get out there—and taking a leap into a completely different world. I also thank you for putting up with my amateur mistakes, not holding them against me, and knowing exactly what to say. To my editor, Kathryn Knigge, I owe you the same gratitude for putting up with my naïveté and helping me navigate this new world of writing, while at the same time, giving me the freedom to say what needs to be said and a platform to share it with the world.

To my husband and son who honored me with support and changed their toothpaste, their eating habits, and their deodorants during this writing process! To my Mom for always being there for me. To my friends and family and early supporters of my work at the JCC and Canyon Ranch, I thank you for your support, your Facebook shares, and listening to my frequent preaching on toxins. I am truly blessed with so many wonderful people in my life.

And to the experts and the change makers who contributed their work and knowledge to this book: Dr. Margaret Cuomo, Anna Castellani, Tammy Fender, Jenefer Palmer, Ellen Gustafson, Dr. Anthony Miller, Ken McAlister, Eileen Fisher, Cynthia Power, and Amy Hall at Eileen Fisher, Jon Wheelan, Robert Tisserand, and the countless others who helped connect me with the right people. Thank you.

INTRODUCTION
How the Story Began

MY JOURNEY to a toxin-free life started twenty years ago.

As the founder of the Good Home Company—a natural products company specializing in "green" cleaning products—I have long been a proponent of a natural, healthy lifestyle. My inspiration for Good Home was my grandparents' farm in Ohio—a place where I spent my childhood summers swimming in the pond, foraging for morels, and eating sweet corn pulled off the stalk in the field. When I first started in 1994, natural cleaning did not exist; Aveda had just taken off and Martha Stewart ruled the airwaves. There was a desire, as there is now, for products that are good for you. Essential oils were being discovered (again), and my love of nature and farm stands inspired me in my own kitchen to create body and home care products over the stove.

So with a few pots and pans, pantry ingredients, and a big dream, the Good Home Company was officially founded on my Grandmother's birthday—September 18—in 1995.

From day one, I created everything by hand (still do for new products) right down to the labels. Each bubble bath and hand cream was made like a pie from scratch, and I personally delivered them to my neighborhood customers in Chelsea. One day—simply out of need—I created a laundry detergent with essential oil of lavender and natural laundry soap. It was an instant hit. Turns out I was not the only one seeking cleaning products that had a recognizable smell and not some made up scent called "orchard." With that one product, we grew by leaps and bounds; awards and press were daily occurrences and a new industry was formed.

This could have been it, and I definitely thought it was my "story" when in fact it was just a chapter.

For someone who had worked twenty years in the natural products category, no one was more surprised than I was when I got the diagnosis almost two years ago of breast cancer. (However, I am pretty sure you could poll anyone who has received a cancer diagnosis, and they will tell you it is *always* shocking).

Although it certainly is not something I ever hope to receive again, for me, cancer was a gift. I was diagnosed extremely early, and after surgery and daily radiation for three months, I was cured. My risk of breast cancer returning is 5 percent or less. Having lost several friends to cancer in their midforties, I felt incredibly fortunate to be a survivor and greeted my daily treatment with joy and appreciation.

When given a life-threatening disease, you are guaranteed to go through some changes and analysis of your person. For me, the lesson was clear; I was being called to share the research I was uncovering and bring awareness on how so many of our day-to-day products are detrimental to our health. Most of us—including me—think that the government does safety checks. Surely everything is tested for its safety to our health and environment; in fact, this couldn't be further from the truth.

In my own industry, we are constantly updating our ingredients as new information comes out. Twenty years ago, we all used parabens as a preservative, and then it was found that they can disrupt your endocrine system. Ten years ago we all used sodium laureth sulfate (SLES), which is a plant-derived chemical that is a common soap synthetic found in everything from detergent to baby wash. However, now it is a known skin irritant and can also be contaminated with 1,4-dioxane—a carcinogen. In 2013, Tide detergent, which used SLS, was reformulated after it was found to be contaminated with more than 60 ppm of 1,4-dioxane. The U.S. government threshold is 25 ppm and less. So thankfully, because of independent testing, this was caught and rectified. But the question remains: If something is known to be a carcinogen, such as 1,4-dioxane, why is it even allowed in our products when we know it caused cancer in laboratory animals? Why doesn't Proctor and Gamble have to test *every* batch of Tide?

Another ingredient of concern, which we have banned from Good Home products, is phthalates. Phthalates are known to disrupt our endocrine system—which monitors everything from metabolism, growth and development, tissue function, sexual function, reproduction, sleep, and mood. If that is the case, then why are they allowed in everything from baby lotion to $300 face creams that we use every single day? Is it any surprise that children are reaching puberty earlier, and women are having a harder time getting pregnant?

Although we are living longer, we are not living healthier. One out of two men and one out of three women will get cancer in their lifetime. This is probably no surprise to you because of the number of diagnoses you see in your own community. Even medical practitioners are concerned with this increase and are calling on government and manufacturers to step up and do their job in protecting us and making sure what they sell us is safe. In her enlightening book and PBS special of the same name, *A World without Cancer*, Dr. Margaret Cuomo (a board-certified radiologist) shares her vast knowledge of this disease and how she sees our constant exposure to these chemical toxins in our daily lives as a definite detriment to our health, impressing on us to demand action from our government and manufacturers to be much more responsible in their regulations and ingredient choices.

The global economy we live in is being led by big businesses creating chemicals, technology, clothing, food, and "beauty" products that are not being tested for their long-term damage to our health; in the meantime, we and our planet are the guinea pigs. The way of the world is to get the product on the market, money in the pocket, and then worry about safety.

There is no reason why anything of harm—to ourselves or to our environment—should be released. Although one would hope that a company has moral values, we know this is not something we can count on, and therefore we need to look to our governments to put our health and wellness before money and growth.

What I find most disturbing is how big businesses alter the facts from consumers for profit. They are selling health, when to the contrary, the ingredients of their products are quite the opposite. The biggest abuser is the food industry, but the beauty industry isn't far behind. The problems are vast but not hopeless. We as consumers have the

power. By refraining from instant gratification and on-demand consumerism, we can change the current landscape. That combined with
putting our health and planet's well-being first—and demanding companies do the same—will indeed make a difference. This altruistic view
is entirely possible and already happening. From larger businesses, like
Eileen Fisher, who repurpose their own clothing into new garments, to
the surge of local farmers' markets selling heirloom vegetables grown
from non-Monsanto seeds, to the rise of artisans creating everything
from skin care to repurposed furniture and finding it in mainstream
stores. It is an inspiring time, and conscious consumerism is a trend that
is definitely being heard. Companies want to meet our demands, and
they will listen and change where they source their ingredients from; so
that organic, non-GMO corn chips you bought are actually helping to
change the world.

Detox Your Home is my journey to a healthier home shared with you.
It is a guidebook to help you examine and absorb, giving you the power
to make the decisions that are right for you and your home. For instance,
vinegar and water may be the cleaning choice for you in your home or
you may be okay with using a soap that is highly processed from coconut
oil. This is not about judgment but about providing you with the information to make your own decisions. Although I do share my opinions
throughout my book, my findings are based on facts and science and
interviews with leaders in their fields of expertise.

It is my belief that you cannot have a healthy home without addressing all parts. Like Eastern religion believes, you must address the individual to heal the whole, so I will share foods that are proven to heal,
bring good health, and should be in your fridge and pantry. We have all
heard the story about mattresses and how they are toxic, that will be covered too. Do you really need to wear an earpiece when talking on your
cell phone (the answer is *yes*) and did you know that one of the biggest
pollutants of our planet is fast fashion? That five-dollar T-shirt at H&M
is extremely harmful in so many ways, and although not affecting your
health directly, it is affecting the health of the worker making it and the
environment your child or their children will live in. I will show you
other choices you have that won't hurt others or the environment.

In his book, *The Third Plate*, Dan Barber, eloquently and passion-
ately, looks at how mass agriculture is poisoning our land and decreasing

the nutritional value of our food. This Michelin Star Chef could "sell out" and continue to capitalize on the farm-to-table concept, but instead he is leading an effort to change the way we see agriculture. An effort that is making a difference. In fact the *New York Times* just reported that major food brands are scrambling to fill the center aisles. Why? Because the message is finally reaching the masses, and we are buying more fresh foods and not buying processed grains and cereals anymore.

This is a new world. We are being called on to change. Our resources are already exhausted and the tank is on red. We, our friends, our family, our neighbors, and our coworkers all know this; it is our leaders and big businesses who don't, but they do see where we spend our money. Every time you shop you are expressing incredible power and the choices you make are directly related to our own health and our planet's; it really is up to you. My job is to give you the knowledge. The more we know, the more we can use that knowledge for the health of ourselves and the future.

Detox Your Home is a compilation of these facts, giving you the power to make that journey to wellness for you, your home, and the planet we call home. Thank you for joining me.

LABELS AND REGULATORS

IN MY WORK, I have found most people have no idea how the products we use and the food we eat is regulated. The time has come for us to be aware. We operate under the assumption that the government is looking out for us and that we do not need to worry. Yes, the government is indeed the watchdog, but sadly it has not restructured or kept up with our rapid industrialization. There are thousands of chemicals on the market that are unregulated because the government does not have the capacity to test them all or the desire to hold back commerce. We have a system that is not proactive; it deals with an issue when something happens.

A great example of this is talc, which has been used in baby powder for years. The family of a deceased woman who died from ovarian cancer (and used talc daily on her genitals), successfully won against a suit against Johnson and Johnson. Talc is mined near asbestos, and although it is supposed to be free of asbestos since 1970, the possibility for cross-contamination exists. It is used in baby powders, cosmetics, such as blushes, eyeshadows, face powders, food, and toothpaste. An article from National Center for Biotechnology Information (NCBI), dated October 2014, discusses how samples of talc from a cosmetic body powder from Italy were proven to have asbestos.[1]

Meanwhile asbestos, which has been known to be a carcinogen since 1970, is *still* on the market in the United States and people *still* die from exposure to it. Although it is no longer manufactured in the United States, it can still be used in the United States in products like roofing and can also still be imported. The United States is not alone in allowing this toxic substance, and the increase of asbestos use has risen dramatically in China, India, Russia, and Brazil.

The problem is how products are regulated. There are guidelines, but most safety concerns are the responsibility of the manufacturer of the product. By giving the manufacturer the control, the safety and health of everyone is in their hands and trust. And as we have experienced, they continue to abuse our trust for profit margins and bonuses. I believe in a world where our elected officials proactively protect our health and well-being over protecting big business, but until that day we must read every label and demand more of the manufacturers.

Here is an extensive list of who regulates our food, cosmetics, cleaners, and our environment in the United States in their *own* words—from their own websites.

REGULATORS

The Environmental Protection Agency (EPA): "The mission of EPA is to protect human health and the environment." The sections they regulate, through information from TSCA, are agriculture, automotive, construction, electric utilities, pesticides, oil and gas, transportation, water (from municipal supplies).

The Toxic Substances Control Act (TSCA): Before leaving office, President Obama signed the Lautenberg Act, a reform to TSCA.

> The Toxic Substances Control Act of 1976 provides the EPA with authority to require reporting, record-keeping and testing requirements, and restrictions relating to chemical substances and/or mixtures. Certain substances are generally excluded from TSCA, including, among others, food, drugs, cosmetics and pesticides.

The U.S. Department of Agriculture (USDA) is responsible for meat, poultry, and vaccines for animal diseases.

The Occupational Safety and Health Administration (OSHA) was created by President Richard Nixon in 1977 and protect U.S. workers from hazardous chemicals and conditions on the job.

The Food and Drug Administration (FDA):

The scope of FDA's regulatory authority is very broad. FDA's responsibilities are closely related to those of several other government agencies. Often frustrating and confusing for consumers is determining the appropriate regulatory agency to contact. The following is a list of traditionally-recognized product categories that fall under FDA's regulatory jurisdiction; however, this is not an exhaustive list.

In general, FDA regulates **foods, drugs, biologics, medical devices, electronic devices that give off radiation, cosmetics, veterinary products, and tobacco products, including:**

- dietary supplements
- bottled water
- food additives
- infant formulas
- other food products (although the USDA plays a lead role in regulating aspects of some meat, poultry, and egg products)
- prescription drugs (both brand-name and generic)
- nonprescription (over-the-counter) drugs
- vaccines
- blood and blood products
- cellular and gene therapy products
- tissue and tissue products
- allergenics
- simple items like tongue depressors and bedpans
- complex technologies such as heart pacemakers
- dental devices
- surgical implants and prosthetics
- microwave ovens
- X-ray equipment
- laser products
- ultrasonic therapy equipment

- mercury vapor lamps
- sunlamps
- color additives found in makeup and other personal care products
- skin moisturizers and cleansers
- nail polish and perfume
- livestock feeds
- pet foods
- veterinary drugs and devices
- cigarettes
- cigarette tobacco
- roll-your-own tobacco
- smokeless tobacco

TSCA monitors toxic chemicals, which then gets reported to the EPA, who in turn protect us from using them and make sure they aren't used. The FDA monitors pretty much everything we use on our body and ingest, except some items such as water and pesticides, where they work with the EPA and then there is meat, which also involves the USDA.

But here is where it gets tricky, on delving in further, this is what the FDA says about cosmetics:

FDA does not approve cosmetics.

Examples of cosmetics are perfumes, makeup, moisturizers, shampoos, hair dyes, face and body cleansers, and shaving preparations.

Cosmetic products and ingredients do not require FDA approval before they go on the market, with one exception: color additives (other than coal tar hair dyes). Cosmetics must be safe for their intended use and properly labeled.

FDA field investigators inspect cosmetic companies, examine imports, and collect samples for analysis. FDA may take action against non-compliant products, or against firms or individuals who violate the law.

And here is what they say about food and supplements:

FDA does not approve dietary supplements.

Unlike new drugs, dietary supplements are not reviewed and approved by FDA based on their safety and effectiveness. Most dietary supplements that contain a new dietary ingredient (a dietary ingredient not marketed in the United States before October 15, 1994) require a notification to FDA seventy-five days before marketing.

The notification must include the information that was the manufacturer or distributor's basis for concluding that the dietary supplement will reasonably be expected to be safe. After dietary supplements are on the market, FDA evaluates their safety through research and adverse event monitoring.

FDA does not approve the food label, including Nutrition Facts.

FDA does not approve individual food labels before food products can be marketed. But FDA regulations require nutrition information to appear on most foods, including dietary supplements. Also, any claims on food products must be truthful and nonmisleading, and must comply with any special requirements for the type of claim.

Manufacturers are required to provide the serving size of the food and information about the nutrient content of each serving on the "Nutrition Facts" panel of the food label (or on the "Supplement Facts" panel for dietary supplements).

And perhaps the most important statement of all is this:

Who is responsible for substantiating the safety of cosmetics?

Companies and individuals who manufacture or market cosmetics have a legal responsibility to ensure the safety of their products. Neither the law nor FDA regulations require specific tests to demonstrate the safety of individual products or ingredients. The law also does not require cosmetic companies to share their safety information with FDA.

What does the FDA approve? They approve drugs. So, while we are busy buying products that are potentially making us sick and not good for us, they are approving pills and other medicines to put a band aid on many illnesses created by lack of good regulations.

SEALS AND LABELS

Because the FDA and EPA are reactionary resources instead of preventative ones, the public has established many watchdog organizations to help protect us. Many of us look to these seals on product labels as assurance that a product is good for us. I am sure they were created with the best of intentions, but they can be misleading and give you the impression something is natural. As their popularity has risen, they have become marketing tools, and although helpful, one must still look at the label and not assume it is all natural. Here is a guide of commonly found seals and what they do and DO NOT mean.

Created by the USDA to regulate the emerging organic market as it grew, the USDA organic seal is one we all look to for our organic produce and now for some makeups and cleaning products (see Figure L.1). But what does it mean? These seals are meant to help us as consumers, but have no doubt, it is also a marketing tool. When I see the organic seal, many things come to mind: a small local farm where no pesticides are used, locally grown in small batches, and a product that is good for me.

In reality, organic food is a huge business, and it most likely is grown on a large farm, probably in California or Mexico and is grown next to conventionally sprayed produce as well. Although Roundup® is not being sprayed, organically grown products can be sprayed with certain natural and synthetic substances. You can find which ones at the following URL: http://blogs.usda.gov/2012/01/25/organic-101-allowed-and-prohibited-substances/. Cross-contamination from their conventionally grown neighbor's farm is a real issue. I found many articles and organizations that help organic farmers protect themselves and their damaged crops, which was encouraging but discouraging as well. Contamination from GMO farms via wind and animals is a real issue, and if we are to remain truly GMO free, this will need to be addressed. Currently the FDA suggests creating a "buffer zone." As an example, the following

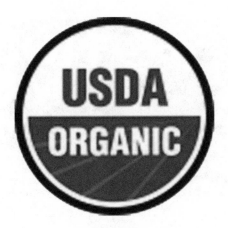

Figure L.1
Source: USDA Organic
(www.organic.org)

URL shows a drawing of one, https://www.ams.usda.gov/sites/default
/files/media/Can%20GMOs%20be%20Used.pdf.

Any product that has the organic seal is also GMO free; however, it is not tested for GMOs and cross-contamination can occur from wind and bird droppings.

To be certified with the USDA organic seal, the product needs to contain 95 percent organic ingredients, excluding water and salt. For a cleaning product that is nearly 95 percent water, that does not amount to much organic. I would much rather use a cleaning product that is non-organic, cleans well, and uses safe ingredients, instead of a cleaning spray filled mostly with water and a few organic essential oils just to meet the guideline and qualify for the organic label. That is marketing. Same with cosmetics. Don't be fooled by a blush that uses organic lavender oil but still contains talc, which can be contaminated with carcinogens.

Carrageen (a concern for digestion) and forms of MSG such as isolates, yeast extracts, and proteins are considered additives and can be added to products with the organic seal.

Lastly, *organic* does not mean an animal led a good life. Organic meats, eggs, butters, and milk come from an animal who was fed a diet of organic grain but still could have lived in a stall all its life and not

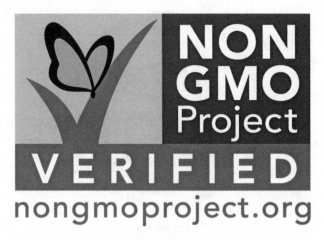

Figure L.2
Source: NON-GMO (www.nongmoproject.org)

roamed the land freely. Look for the label that states "raised humane," which regulates the quality of life for animals used for food.

The Non-GMO Project Verified seal is now found on many products out of need because the U.S. government is still debating the idea whether mandatory GMO labeling should occur (see Figure L.2). Until they decide, food manufacturers can get approved for several non-GMO seals; I chose this one because it is the most widely recognized. Although the organic seal should technically mean non-GMO free as well, testing for contamination is not specifically required, but it may be done as part of the 5 percent testing requirement under the USDA organic certification process or when contamination is suspected.

The Non-GMO Project states on their website that, "To meet the Non-GMO Project Standard, an ingredient derived from a high-risk organism will need test results from the raw source material to prove that it is non-GMO. Testing of risk ingredients is done at critical points in the supply chain to verify that GMO contamination is below the applicable action threshold."[2]

Their thresholds for GMO contamination are as follows:

- Seed and other propagation materials: 0.25%[3]
- Human food and products ingested or used directly on skin: 0.9%

- Cleaning products, textiles, and products not ingested or used directly on skin: 1.5%
- Animal feed and supplements: 5%

This seal does *not* mean it is free of spraying of pesticides or glyphosate (Roundup). It does not mean it is "100% GMO free." This label can also apply to cosmetic and cleaning products.

The top GMO crops and their percentages in the United States are:

- 94% of soybeans
- 93% of cotton
- 92% of corn (This is field corn grown to feed animals, which in turn we eat. Monsanto just introduced a GMO sweet corn though.)
- 70% of squash
- 77% of papaya
- 90% of Canola (rapeseed) plants
- 60% of sugar beets

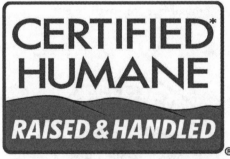

CERTIFIED* HUMANE RAISED & HANDLED

* Meets the Humane Farm Animal Care Program standards, Which include nutritious diet without antibiotics, or hormones, animals raised with shelter, resting areas, sufficient space and the ability to engage in natural behaviors.

Figure L.3
Source: CERTIFIED HUMANE
(www.certifiedhumane.org)

Certified Humane is a food label that is meant to inform you that the animal that you are eating or the food it provided in eggs, milk, and so on, was treated humanely (see Figure L.3). You can see their site for complete details. In summary, the animal was raised without antibiotics or hormones, with proper shelter and not put in cages, crates, or tie stalls. Chickens must be able to flap their wings and take dust baths (this is not usually the case in most chicken farms where they are packed in tight), and pigs must be allowed to roam and root. Their diet must be free of hormones, antibiotics, and animal by-products. The Humane Farm Animal Care program was written by a forty-member scientific committee and covers all aspects of husbandry from birth through slaughter and supports each animal's ability to engage in its natural behaviors.

It does not mean the food is organic, and organic doesn't mean the food was raised humanely.

These two logos shown in Figures L.4 and L.6 can be found on cosmetics or cleaning products. It certifies that the product and its ingredients are free of any animal by-products. This includes dye made from crushed insects, honey and beeswax produced by bees, lanolin from sheep wool, or glycerin from animal fat. It also certifies that the product and the ingredients were not tested on animals. It does not mean the product is organic, chemical free, or toxin free.

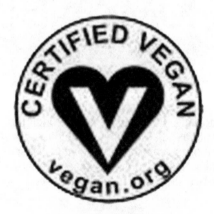

Figure L.4
Source: VEGAN (www.vegan.org)

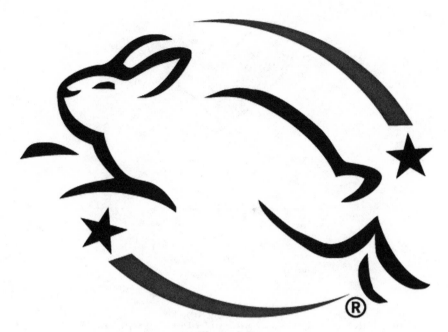

Figure L.5
Source: LEAPING BUNNY (www.leapingbunny.org)

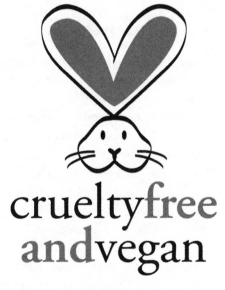

Figure L.6
Source: PETA (www.peta.org)

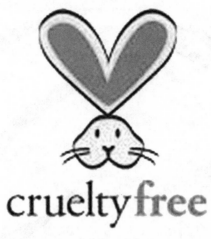

Figure L.7
Source: PETA (www.peta.org)

These logos in Figures L.5 and L.7 appear on products (cosmetics and household) that were not tested on animals. This includes ingredients as well. It does not mean it is vegan (free of animal by-products), and it does not mean it is organic, natural, chemical free, or toxin free.

INGREDIENTS

There are many resources on the Web right now trying to do the overwhelming task of data banking every single chemical ingredient used in cleaning, personal care, and beauty products. Although I commend them, there are many factors one needs to take into consideration, including how it is being used or applied and how much of the ingredient is in it. Synthetic perfumes, for example, often get bad grades, but not all synthetic perfumes are "bad." It is true that phthalates are often found in these man-made perfumes, but not every perfume has them. If a company wants to use a higher-grade perfume free of toxins, they can. It just costs more, and like most of what we will discuss in this book, money is a driver in most of the toxins in our home.

For instance, my company uses man-made fragrances that are completely phthalate free and benzene free. Synthetic perfumes can contain benzenes, but so do some essential oils. That is why it is so important to look at each formula, and unfortunately, this is not done. There are millions of products and thousands of ingredients to cover, so algorithms are often used in lieu of product testing, giving false and sometimes detrimental information. In addition, many of the sites also have their own seal, which manufacturers pay for. This in turn creates a conflict of interest and brings money to the table, which sadly begins to corrupt what is supposed to be a public service.

Where should one go for honest information? Good question. A simple Google search on sodium lauryl sulfate (SLS) will have many alarming results; however, one must look at the resource and do many searches before reaching a conclusion. I look at Material Safety Data Sheets (MSDS), which can leave out information and are not always reliable, so I check several. I also like to look at government websites from all countries and research documents. Surprisingly the U.S. government has many studies available, that if you take the time to read thoroughly, you can draw your own conclusions. The Centers for Disease Control and Prevention (CDC) has informational studies when it comes to disease prevention. One that many refer to is the use of essential oil of lemon eucalyptus instead of DEET, because it was found that lemon eucalyptus was as effective.

Some consumer websites, such as ewg.org, have a large catalog of MSDS and research, but much of it is outdated or not updated on new findings, and their grading of overall products uses an algorithm that does not consider percentage levels, which is crucial in determining safety.

The answer is there is no answer. It is up to us to find trusted resources and do our own research. I take a personal approach and like to know who grows my food, makes my clothes, and creates the products I put on my body. The resurgence of handmade, artisan goods is wonderful for our economy and for our health. I will share my resources with you, but I encourage you to meet your local farmer and buy your produce, meat, and dairy products form a local grower/farm. Shop Etsy and look for artists at flea markets and local bazaars who you can talk to about ingredients and see their ethics firsthand.

The more we ask, the more companies will listen and comply. In 1995 when I started, no one listed their ingredients on cleaning products, and now if you don't, you are the anomaly. Your requests to companies to clean up their act is absolutely being heard; we are only powerless when we take no action on our own behalf.

HOW TO READ A LABEL

If the manufacturer is honest, a label is your best friend. In the beauty and personal care industry, you must list your ingredients. In the cleaning industry, you do not, unless the product makes a claim and is an over-the-counter (OTC) drug like hand sanitizer. If a cosmetic makes a claim, for example, sunscreen, it is considered an OTC as well.

Ingredients are supposed to be listed in order of quantity, with the largest amount starting first. This is for cosmetics and food. The ingredients for Jergens Skin Firming Daily Toning Moisturizer that follow start with water. This is the predominate ingredient. It ends with hydrolyzed elastin and is the ingredient that is used the least in this lotion. In looking at this lotion, the first five ingredients are liquid and oil that make the cream; it is petroleum (think Vaseline) and water blended. Cetearyl alcohol is not a cosmetic cocktail, but a solid fatty ingredient derived from petroleum or palm oil—probably petroleum because that is cheaper—and is used to thicken products. It is also found in food. The other stuff added in the middle are preservatives, DMDM Hydantoin specifically is a preservative that works by releasing formaldehyde—a carcinogen.

INGREDIENTS: WATER, GLYCERIN, CETEARYL ALCO-HOL, PETROLATUM, MINERAL OIL, CETEARETH-20, ALUMINUM STARCH OCTENYLSUCCINATE, CYCLO-PENTASILOXANE, ACRYLATES COPOLYMER, DIMETHI-CONE, STEARIC ACID, GLYCERYL DILAURATE, DMDM HYDANTOIN, METHYLPARABEN, FRAGRANCE, BUTY-LENE GLYCOL, ACRYLATES/C10-30 ALKYL ACRYLATE CROSSPOLYMER, PROPYLPARABEN, HYDROLYZED WHEAT PROTEIN/PVP CROSSPOLYMER, SODIUM HYDROXIDE, ARGININE, TOCOPHERYL ACETATE, CENTELLA ASIAT-ICA EXTRACT, COCOS NUCIFERA (COCONUT) WATER,

HYDROLYZED COLLAGEN, POLYIMIDE-1, WITHANIA SOMNIFERA ROOT EXTRACT, FUCUS VESICULOSUS EXTRACT, HYDROLYZED ELASTIN

For food labels, the same theory applies: the first ingredient is what was mostly used to make the product and the last ingredient is in it the least. The label that follows is from Oreos. The first ingredient is unbleached enriched flour. The stuff in parentheses are what is in the flour. The second ingredient in this cookie is sugar. Anything in parentheses is an ingredient in that ingredient.

INGREDIENTS: UNBLEACHED ENRICHED FLOUR (WHEAT FLOUR, NIACIN, REDUCED IRON, THIAMINE MONONITRATE {VITAMIN B1}, RIBOFLAVIN {VITAMIN B2}, FOLIC ACID), SUGAR, PALM, AND/OR CANOLA OIL, COCOA (PROCESSED WITH ALKALI), HIGH FRUCTOSE CORN SYRUP, LEAVENING (BAKING SODA, AND/OR CALCIUM PHOSPHATE), CORNSTARCH, SALT, SOY LEC-ITHIN, VANILLIN—AN ARTIFICIAL FLAVOR, CHOCO-LATE. CONTAINS WHEAT, SOY.

So now that we know how to read a label, let's begin our look at deciphering what's in these products.

PART I

DETOX YOUR SKIN

THIS SECTION will most likely be the hardest to make a change in. I know it was for me. When I went through all my products, I was shocked at the number of chemicals I was putting on my skin daily with makeup alone. Thanks to advertising and TV, we are truly under pressure to look a certain way. Health and aging naturally is unfortunately not the popular look, and the pressure to wear makeup and have a certain body shape and hair color is immense. I also think this is one area where most of us put blinders on. Many, including health professionals, are willing to take the risk for short-term benefits. Botox is a great example; millions of people regularly inject a poison into their skin for a few short months of no wrinkles. Never mind the problems that will come twenty years down the road.

As we all know, billions are spent by manufacturers to convince us that a face cream, body moisturizer, or whitening paste will bring us the youth our society seems to covet. Unfortunately, most of the ingredients are chemical creations from petroleum, often with the addition of harmful endocrine disrupters such as phthalates. Skin creams, body lotions, shower gels, bubble baths, scrubs, and so on all fall under the FDA's supervision, *but* they do not require FDA approval to be placed on the shelf and sold. FDA approval is only required if you are making a claim, such as that it reduces wrinkles by 10 percent, kills germs, and so on. Because creams, soaps, and lotions make no claims, the rules they fall under are minimal. Font size, directions, the amount of product, and where it is manufactured are all required. Ingredients fall under good manufacturing process (GMP), leaving it entirely up to the manufacturer to create a clean, safe product that is indeed good for the wearer.

All manufacturers, including myself, rely on the chemists and developers of our products to create with ingredients that are healthy and without any long-term effects. The chemists are equally reliant on TSCA to determine if a chemical is safe. But the issue is that chemicals are being introduced before proper testing is done.

Not knowing what on the market now is toxic should have us all protesting in front of the White House. It is hard to understand how we can increase our technology by leaps and bounds, and yet we have not found a way to test a chemical for safety before releasing it on the market. This seems to be the way, and I hope with this book and the many others out there that we will someday have a government that puts our health first.

Until then, we will need to be diligent and constantly check as new ingredients are approved. An example of this is in preservatives. A new preservative, Japanese Honeysuckle, is being touted as a natural way to preserve many skin care products. It is an extract from the honeysuckle flower that also mimics a synthetic paraben. It has a benzene ring in its structure, which is a concern because all parabens (known to disrupt your endocrine system) have the same structure. By being a potential paraben, it also has the ability to mimic human estrogen like synthetic parabens do, and an increase in estrogen is a cause for certain types of breast cancer. This is now a widely used preservative in many natural skin care products and has not been approved by the FDA. If you have paraben allergies, you will also be allergic to the Japanese Honeysuckle preservative as well. Confused yet? You are not alone.

In writing this book, there are many rabbit holes I went down and could have gone down with blog after blog. There are many sites that try to provide the consumer with help and guidance on products that are indeed safe, but the fact is even their algorithms are far from perfect. For me, I have scaled back my beauty regime significantly and would rather go with simple than with a bunch of products that "may" be okay. I limit myself to the facts and ingredients that are either 100 percent natural or I make my own.

Sustainably speaking, I now use maybe one-fourth of the products I once used. Not only has this reduced my yearly trash footprint, but it has been liberating to reduce my grooming routine substantially and just focus on cleaning and treating my skin and hair with health—not focusing on what I don't have or need to improve (i.e., longer lashes, bigger eyes, bouncier hair) but rather caring for what I do have—a healthy body.

As with most things, we need to consider the long term, before buying into the short term. I also think if we can look at beauty products as food for our skin, we will be less likely to apply unnatural dyes and ingredients to it daily. And fortunately, as the desire for healthier products increase, the industry is responding. Every year there are much better options to groom yourself with healthy ingredients that work. I will share with you the companies I have uncovered in my research and their products that are hopefully going to be the new standard for beauty.

CHAPTER 1

FACE AND BODY CREAMS

MOST BODY LOTIONS and face creams on the shelves are chemicals and derived from petroleum (crude oil sludge). You will find that some good things are thrown in there in small amounts, but most of the products on the shelves are petroleum oil and water with a few added vitamins.

Everything you put on your skin is absorbed into your bloodstream to some degree—depending on the ingredient, application, molecular composition, and so on. If something is put on your body day after day after day, it can build up. In fact, parabens, which are a common preservative in thousands of brands, are found in the breast tissue of women with breast cancer, and I would suspect would be found in the tissue of all of us if we had some removed. I am not saying they cause cancer, but I do want to know why they are found in our bodies and phthalates are found in our urine.

I do not have enough pages to list everything, but what follows are several common ingredients in skin care and body care products that you should know about. To investigate further, www.safecosmetics.org does a good job policing ingredients and is worth bookmarking.

PRESERVATIVES

Anything with water requires a preservative for an extended shelf life. Preservatives are important because a person with a compromised immune system can become ill if a poorly preserved product growing bacteria is used. However, as much as they help, they also have huge concerns. I hope that the twenty-first century finds us with a broad-spectrum preservative for skin care we can trust, is natural, and is not harmful. Until then, we are trading off elmination of bacteria growth for severe allergies, endocrine disruption, and formaldehyde exposure.

Some preservatives smell good too, and perfumers use them in creating a fragrance. Because fragrance ingredients are numerous and are not required to be listed, you may end up using a product with a preservative you are allergic or sensitive to without even knowing it.

I wish I had recommendations for natural preservatives, but there aren't any that provide a broad spectrum, which is needed for products containing water. There are many products being developed, but their market safety is not well established and I am hesitant to recommend anything without five years of good testing. Some natural preservatives combine natural and synthetic ingredients that they sell under a brand name like Germoben. For those of us who want to know exactly what is in the product, this makes our label reading all the more difficult.

There are about five commonly used preservatives in cosmetics. Here is a snapshot of some and their effects on our health.

Parabens

- Common names include butylparaben, methylparaben, propyl paraben, or any ingredient with a "paraben" at the end.

Impact on Your Health

Parabens are known endocrine disruptors. Your endocrine system (see Figure 1.1) controls everything from puberty to your weight to sexual function. All anyone needs to do is look at the rising rates of infertility and children reaching puberty younger and younger and a huge red flag should go up. Just like the patches you put on to quit smoking, the creams you put on your skin are also absorbed into your bloodstream. What that exact amount is varies on the molecular size, which depends on the product and ingredient; however even if it is the tiniest amount,

ENDOCRINE SYSTEM

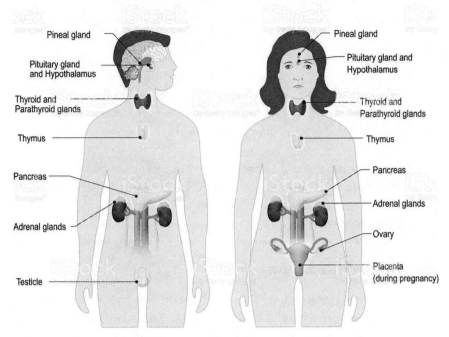

Figure 1.1
Source: ISTOCK IMAGE 524015138

the buildup is significant. Most of us have large amounts of parabens in our bodies. For something that is supposed to be innocuous, it does not appear to be so.

In addition to our skin care products, we are exposed to parabens daily in our food. According to a study done in Albany, parabens are quite prevalent in pancake syrup, jellies, pickles, and even fish.[1]

Impact on the Environment

In all the data I pored over, I could not find conclusive information on this. Some sources say it is biodegradable, and others say no. I did find that parabens are prevalent in our drinking water. This would lead me to believe that no, it is not biodegradable. It is dumped through our water system at such high levels via shampoos, detergents, foods, and pesticides and although not monitored, independent studies have found it there. So much so, that the state of Minnesota put the following out in 2011.

> How much propyl paraben is in Minnesota water?
> MDH believes propyl paraben might be a common contaminant in water because it is widely used. However, there is no information about levels in Minnesota waters.[2]

In my opinion the use of parabens is something we all need to eliminate. It is clear we all have it built up in our bodies, and before we keep using them, we need to look at the full effects of this build up in our bodies and the harms.

Methylisothiazolinone (MIT)

- Common names include 2-methyl-4-isothiazoline-3-one, Neolone 950 preservative, MI, OriStar MIT, Microcare MT, Methylchloroisothiazolinone (CMIT): 5-Chloro-2-methyl-4-isothiazolin-3-one, and MCI.

Impact on Your Health

This preservative is currently being looked at by the European Union (EU) as one that should not be used in skin care products that are left on. Many are highly allergic to it and get severe redness if they use a product containing it. As with all preservatives, it is recommended at low levels; however if you have a severe sensitivity to it, any amount is too much. There are also findings showing neurotoxicity in animals.[3]

Here is advice from the Dermatitis Society from an article in the *New York Times*:

> The dermatitis society named MI its "allergen of the year" in 2013, a listing intended to give attention to problematic and often obscure substances. That same year, the Scientific Committee on Consumer

Safety, a European advisory group, said that MI should be used only in limited quantities for rinse-off products, like soaps and shampoos, and that "no safe concentrations" existed for leave-on products like lotions.[4]

The EPA has MIT on their list as something workers need to be protected from. It is found in skin care and in paints, solvents and other industrial products.

If this is in a leave-on skin care product, I would stay away for allergy reasons alone. Unfortunately, it is often hidden.

Impact on the Environment

This preservative has been found to be toxic to fish.

Phenoxyethanol

- Common names include 2-Phenoxyethanol, Euxyl K® 400 (mixture of Phenoxyethanol and 1,2-dibromo-2,4-dicyanobutane), and PhE.

Impact on Your Health

Phenoxyethanols affect the nervous system. In 2008, the FDA banned Mommy's Bliss Nipple Cream because phenoxyethanol, found in the cream, was depressing the central nervous system and causing vomiting and diarrhea in breast-feeding infants. Phenoxyethanols are sometimes hidden in preservative blends with caprylhydroxamic acid. They are also found in most fragrances because they have an aroma perfumers like to use. Unfortunately, if it is in a perfume, it won't be listed on the label. To avoid it, make sure to use products that are fragrance free. It is not good in anything topical, and it is also in the top list of chemicals that cause allergic reactions.

Impact on the Environment

This preservative does not have any that I could find.

2-bromo-2-nitropropane-1,3-diol, Diazolidinyl urea

- Common names include Imidazolidinyl urea, DMDM hydantoin, Hydroxymethylglycinate, Quaternium-15, and Trishydroxymethyl-nitromethane.

Impact on Your Health

Commonly used in cosmetics but also found in face, body, and dental products, these preservatives are known formaldehyde releasers. Formaldehyde is a carcinogen. Although 0.5 percent of formaldehyde is allowed in products in the United States and EU, I am not sure they considered daily use, day after day, year after year. No reason to even include them when there are other options.

Impact on the Environment

Tris(hydroxymethyl)nitromethane is toxic to fish, and 2-bromo-2-nitropropane-1,3-diol is toxic to fish and releases toxic gases if burned.

Sodium Benzoate and Potassium Sorbate

Impact on Your Health

Probably the least harmful preservatives, but not without concerns. Neither are great preventers of bacteria and need to be used together or with another preservative to ensure a product is properly preserved. Sodium benzoate turns into a benzene—a carcinogen—when combined with vitamin C (an ingredient commonly found in skin creams, lotions, and body washes) in liquid drinks.[5] I could not find any studies on this with cosmetics, which I find concerning. I would make sure vitamin C is not present when sodium benzoate is.

Potassium sorbate is relatively harmless and just does not prevent bacteria growth over a longer period of time.

Use products that use these as a preservative within three to six months.

Impact on the Environment

Sodium benzoate has been shown to biodegrade 97 percent in twenty-eight days with minimal bioaccumulation.[6] Potassium sorbate was shown to biodegrade by 75 percent in twenty-eight days and have minimal bioaccumulation.[7]

Caprylhydroxamic Acid

Impact on Your Health

This gentle and natural preservative derived from coconut oil looks good, but it is often sold as a blend with phenoxyethanol and methylpropanediol to be more effective. Unfortunately, companies do not always disclose this. If the top three ingredients include water and the only preservative is caprylhydroxamic acid, call and check to make sure before using.

Impact on the Environment

Carpylhydoxamic acid has no impact that I could find.

Japanese Honeysuckle (*Ioniceria japonica*) and Essential Oils

Impact on Your Health

Japanese Honeysuckle is the newest "natural' preservative. Marketed under the name "Plantservative," there are some controversies surrounding it. First its molecular structure is similar to parabens—not identical; however, it does have a benzene ring and anything with a benzene ring has the potential of being an endocrine disruptor. There have also been contamination rumors with this preservative. It does contain chemical parabens, or rather, companies are omitting that they are also add parabens to the Japanese Honeysuckle. There are concerns as to its effectiveness as a preservative as well. If using it, make sure it has been tested independently for contamination.

Essential oils can provide short-term preservative help but no more than a month's time. They simply are not effective enough to preserve a product with a high water content. Extracts such as grape seed or grape-fruit seed extracts have also been shown to regularly be contaminated with other preservatives, which is another example of why we should not allow manufacturers to self-regulate. If you are making your own products at home and use them within a few weeks and are careful to store them out of sunlight and in the refrigerator, then I would feel comfortable with an essential oil preservative but not for anything that needs a shelf life.

Impact on the Environment

Japanese honeysuckle has no impact that I could find.

How to Detox

I wish it were as simple as using a product within a week's time, but for many of us, this is highly unrealistic. We need to develop safer, less harmful preservatives for multiple uses. One preservative does not cover all products or contaminants, and it may prevent growth in a skin cream, but not in a body lotion. Here are a few suggestions on how to buy skin care products with minimal exposure to preservatives.

1. Use a product that does not contain water. Facial oils, body oils, and anything without water do not need to be preserved with as strong a preservative as one with water. Water is the first ingredient to grow bacteria, so if you want to be 100 percent preservative free, use oils such as coconut, olive, jojoba, and sesame on your body and to moisturize. I use jojoba as an eye makeup remover, and coconut oil to moisturize my body.
2. If using a water-based product like a toner, a bit of alcohol can preserve it. You don't want to use pure alcohol on your face; however I make a rose water toner for my skin that uses distilled water and a little witch hazel, which has a percentage of alcohol in it already. Alcohol is also the reason perfumes do not need preservatives.
3. Use products that require refrigeration. There are a few small brands out there who make cosmetics to order and refrigerate them. This will last as long as food.

4. Use products with a higher pH level. pH levels can require less of a preservative because a higher pH level means bacteria are less likely to grow.

I use creams with sodium benzoate and potassium sorbate, taking care that vitamin C or citrus oils are not in them. Oils are now my preferred moisturizer and a jar of organic coconut oil can be used on your hair, face, and body. Because most of our personal care and cosmetics fall under best business practices, we must look for sources we can trust and who have testing practices in place.

ADVICE FROM THE EXPERTS

Besides making my own, there are two brands in my skin care routine I am faithful to. I have yet to find anything comparable, and you will hear me espousing their incredible products. Both Tammy Fender and Jenefer Palmer are truly motivated by the healing powers of natural ingredients and are committed to this path.

A jar of their cream will last three months and when you factor that in, the cost is the same, but so much better than the drugstore petroleum cream you are buying for twenty-five dollars. They also work. That can't always be said for natural products.

We must start understanding that what we put on our skin is as important as what we put in our body, and by using products like Tammy's and Jenefer's, it will make the switch to natural not only easy but also life changing.

Q-and-A with Jenefer Palmer, Founder of Osea, www.oseamalibu.com

Q: Why should we use natural products? We all want to look young and beautiful as we grow older. Shouldn't I use the technology available even if it is a chemical? What is the harm?

A: Lab-created, synthetic skin care products entice us with promises of radical results, but often at the cost of our overall health and the health of the environment. As a spa director, I quickly learned that synthetic ingredients can irritate your skin, clog pores, and may cause conditions such as eczema and dermatitis. I even discovered that many skincare products contain compounds that are potentially hazardous to health, such as parabens and phthalates (both hormone disrupters), petroleum (a by-product of the oil refinery process) and polyethylene glycols (PEGs) (known carcinogens)—just to name a few.

Q: Why natural? What is the benefit? Do they work as well?

A: When it comes to skin care, I've always believed that transformational results shouldn't involve compromise. Natural, organic products can deliver the same—if not better—results than their synthetic counterparts. For every synthetic ingredient claiming to produce a radical skin-changing outcome, there is an equally effective natural alternative. Instead of using toxic skin-brightening agents, we use undaria algae, Japanese matsutake mushroom, and bearberry leaf to naturally brighten the skin and ease hyperpigmenation. As an alternative to retinol and benzoyl peroxide (used in acne treatments), we found macrocystis algae, tea tree, cypress, and thyme essential oils to be highly effective in treating blemish-prone skin without causing dryness or peeling. In place of synthetic alpha hydroxy acids, we use grapefruit essential oil and lactic acid (derived from fermented beets) to exfoliate and reveal soft, younger-looking skin. I'm a huge fan of saccharomyces extracts, which are natural peptides derived from yeast cells that plump and revitalize skin. Our renowned bioavailable seaweed concentrates stimulate collagen production and deeply hydrate skin. In my journey with OSEA, I am continuously discovering that when you feed your skin with all of nature's miraculous superfoods, you actually eliminate the need for synthetic ingredients entirely.

Q: Why are ingredients from the sea so good for us?

A: The healing benefits of the sea are endless. Seaweed (or marine algae) is one of the most abundant sources of vitamins, minerals, amino acids, antioxidants, and essential fatty acids. It is actually far richer in trace elements than land plants! Seaweed is unique in that it contains bioavailable ingredients, meaning that its active compounds are more readily absorbed by your body. Greater absorption of nutrients means better results for your skin. Because of its bioavailable nature, seaweed provides a myriad of natural antiaging and anti-inflammatory benefits including calming redness, healing acne, brightening, hydrating, mineralizing, and boosting collagen production.

Q: How does OSEA Malibu maintain quality? Our oceans are polluted; is it still safe to use ingredients from them?

A: Source really does matter. We source our gigartina, undaria, and macrocystis algae from the most pristine waters in the world. Our seaweed originates from the Sea of Patagonia, at the confluence of the southward-flowing Brazil current and the Antarctic Circumpolar current. These frigid waters and constantly shifting extremes of sea surface temperature help to produce the world's most bioavailable, nutrient-rich seaweed. OSEA's seaweed is eco-responsibly hand-foraged as it naturally makes its way to the shores. I am also very proud that our seaweed species have the unique distinction of being USDA certified organic.

Q: What are your favorite super ingredients for the skin?

A: I absolutely love gigartina algae; it makes your skin feel amazing and is the key ingredient in almost all of our products. It helps to stimulate collagen and even protects skin from pollution! In its natural seawater environment, gigartina is exposed to UV [ultraviolet] sunlight and harsh climate conditions. It is able to repair and regenerate its own cells, thanks to its rich content of polysaccharides, antioxidants, and DNA-repairing enzymes. Gigartina offers this same incredible protection against environmental aggressors to your skin.

Q-and-A with Tammy Fender, Founder, www. tammyfender.com

Q: Many women like the idea of natural, but are afraid it won't "work." They will use chemicals to prevent wrinkles to their detriment. What are your experiences with this and how can this mind-set be changed?

A: Practicing holistic medicine, we don't treat wrinkles, but serve each person as a whole, and on every level—physically, but also emotionally, mentally, and spiritually. The beauty industry is full of quick-fix fads, but long-term, lasting results come from consistent holistic care, revealing a deep beauty that shines from within. Slow beauty is the real thing—and it can take three to six months for clients to transform. Habitual patterns make all the difference; from what we eat to how we manage stress throughout the day.

Q: What concerns/issues do you see in your daily work from customers using fillers, Botox, and other toxins to be more beautiful and younger?

A: The question I'm most often asked is "How can I slow the aging process?" While many chemical antiaging techniques may actually damage skin, my collection harnesses the Pure Living Energy© of ancient botanical remedies in order to stimulate new cell growth, protect the skin from environmental factors, support resiliency and elasticity while replenishing skin with ultra-concentrated nutrients and hydration.

Q: If you could speak to every woman in this world, what would you urge them to use and what would you urge them *not* to use?

A: The skin is our body's largest organ, and it is designed to protect us from whatever does not belong inside the body. The skin rejects potential toxins—including petrochemicals, paragons, and synthetic compounds—and the results can be redness or irritation and can even precipitate medical issues. When we recognize that what we put onto the skin is just as important as what we eat, it creates a shift. Our bodies can perfectly process—and so truly benefit from—the pure essences of plants, which are loaded with oxygen and vital nutrients, and can pass quickly through the tissues to deliver everything we need at the cellular level.

Q: What is your favorite ingredient that every woman should have in their beauty cabinet?

A: Pure essence of rose is one of my favorite medicinal remedies for skin. It has miraculous rejuvenating qualities, enhancing cellular growth, but it also has the highest vibration of all the essences, allowing a sense of peace to envelop the heart center.

Q: What is your process in developing a product and how do you make such wonderful and effective creams and serums without the use of chemicals?

A: I work hands-on in my apothecary, which is my passion. While years of research goes into every blend, there is also an intuitive harmony at work, and somehow each combination feels like it simply could not be any other way. Ancient and sacred remedies from the botanical world are incredibly potent—I love to work with these powerful healing elements every day.

Q: Do you see a direct link to food and environmental toxins and our skin? Is there a way to reverse this? (I have changed my skin through your products and a vegetarian diet!)

A: Skin is very resilient—it takes time—but using pure, holistic formulas, we can reverse the effects of toxins on skin, especially when supported by holistic lifestyle choices. Revealing our true radiance might mean making certain dietary changes, for example, in choosing pure, organic foods, or in eating foods in their most natural, raw state, or in consuming less inflammatory foods. These choices shine in the vibrant glow they bring to skin.

PHTHALATES

Many have heard of phthalates, but are unsure of what they actually are. Phthalates are a filler ingredient added to perfumes, lotions, shampoos, nail polish, and plastics. They make plastics more flexible, and in personal care products they control viscosity and keep products from separating (i.e., an emulsifier). Phthalates have been shown to affect the reproduction system of animals. Like parabens, they are an endocrine disruptor. The CDC tested the urine of 2,636 or more participants ages six years and older, and every one had phthalates in their system, women more so than men (women generally use more lotions, hairsprays, and cosmetics). Many target fragrance as the issue because it can be a part of a fragrance blend, but this is just the tip of the iceberg. Phthalates are found in plastic water bottles, food containers, IV tubes, shower curtains, rain coats, rain boots, your car, nail polish, insect repellant, and even dairy products because cows are milked by phthalate laden plastic tubes. They are unavoidable, but you must try to limit them for your health. In skin care products, only buy those labeled as "phthalate-free." Not all fragrances have phthalates (Good Home does not), and if you want to be sure, call the company. A product could be fragrance-free and still have phthalates. I am absolutely convinced that the increase of phthalates in our lives via packaging and ingredients is causing a host of health issues—including reproductive issues—that are so prevalent today. Avoid them as much as you can. Always call and ask the company their stance because they are not listed on products. Also, write to your congressional representative and ask for all products containing phthalates to be labeled as such.

The chemical names for phthalates, although rarely listed, are DEP, DBP, and DEHP.

Impact on Your Health

Some of the effects of phthalates are reproduction issues, infertility, weight gain, depression, miscarriage, genital deformity in boys, hormone disruptor, asthma in children, birth defects, and breast cancer.

Impact on the Environment

Our water, air, and food contain phthalates. More than 11 billion pounds of phthalates are produced worldwide every year.

How to Detox

Only use skin care that certifies they are phthalate-free. Many label it now, and if they don't, write them and ask. If there is a fragrance in your product, you really must make sure it is phthalate-free because it can be "hidden" in there. Avoid soft plastics and cheap drug store brands, which are huge culprits of using phthalates.

Two research studies you should read with regard to phthalates are:

- "Environmental phthalate exposure in relation to reproductive outcomes and other health endpoints in humans," from *Environmental Research*[8] and
- "Biological impact of phthalates," from *Toxicology Letters*.[9]

CREAM BASES AND OILS

One of the biggest crimes in lotions and creams are the bases being used. Most creams—high end too—are using a petroleum derivative. Mineral oil, petrolatum, and paraffin all come from crude oil. The drilling of oil creates a sludge around the pipes and the men who were drilling it discovered that it kept their hands soft. And that is how Vaseline was born.

Although there are concerns with possible 1,4 dioxane contamination during the manufacturing process, there are no ill health effects from mineral oil that I could find. But its environmental effects are huge. A derivative of crude oil, it is one part of our reliance on oil. It is a cheap, plentiful ingredient that gives the appearance of softer skin by creating a barrier on top of it. In other words, your skin literally cannot breathe. It is like putting an airtight plastic lid on top of it.

My other issue is cost. There are many high-end creams out there, including one famous one that sells for $300 a jar, and they are primarily cheap, mineral oil. Although they may add some sea algae and other minerals and natural ingredients, that product is 80 percent mineral oil. You might as well buy a jar of Vaseline or Aquaphor and put it on your face.

I avoid petroleum products and use shea butter, coconut oil, jojoba oil, and other natural oils with living plant ingredients to bring vitamins and health to my skin, and not the after-sludge of a product I put in my car or heat my home with.

Petroleum (Mineral Oil and Petrolatum)

Impact on Your Health

There is possible contamination from manufacturing with 1,4-dioxane (classified carcinogen).

Impact on the Environment

This is a by-product of crude oil and increases our dependency to it. The production of oil is a significant contributor to greenhouse gas emissions, which increase climate change.

How to Detox

Use a cream whose base is shea butter, coconut oil, olive oil, jojoba, avocado, or another plant-based option. Mineral oil is not needed and is just a cheap alternative to natural.

Emulsifiers

When you combine an oil and a liquid, you will need an emulsifier to keep the product from eventually separating. Common ones are PEGs and propylene glycol, also known as 1,2-dihydroxypropane, 1,2-propanediol, methyl glycol, and trimethyl glycol. These chemicals do a few things; they bind the water and oil together and also are an emollient. Propylene glycol is also used in your car as an antifreeze. I have seen it used as the second ingredient (basically the product base) in $120 face creams.

PEGs are also used to help penetrate the skin (make it softer, more pliable); so if crappy ingredients are used, which they usually are if they are using PEGs, then the crap is getting into your skin easier. PEGs are followed by numbers (e.g., PEG-20, PEG-100, and often combined with another molecule like stearate). The number is the molecule size, and the higher the number, the smaller the particle and more penetration into the epidermis.

These two ingredients are basically used to make a cream look smooth and silky, help ingredients penetrate the skin and are also gooey and soft like silicone and give your skin a softer feel.

The problem is they are often contaminated with other ingredients that are carcinogens such as 1,4-dioxane and ethylene oxide and heavy metals, which will also be going into your skin.

Impact on Your Health

PEGs are not the concern. The concern is the possible contamination of carcinogens, ethylene oxide and 1,4-dioxane, that happens when making them. They are also known to be skin irritants and may cause sensitization.

Impact on the Environment

PEGs are found in our water via all the personal care products that contain them.

How to Detox

Use products that use natural softeners and emulsifiers like vegetable glycerin, beeswax, lecithin, candelilla wax, and acacia wax.

CHAPTER 2

SHAMPOOS, SOAPS, AND CONDITIONERS

NEXT OUR daily bathing will be explored. The soaps we will look at are liquid. Most liquid soaps are not actually soaps at all, but a chemical derivative of petroleum oil. They are cheap and abundant and do absolutely nothing to make your skin healthier. The worst part is that many of these chemical ingredients cause drying of the skin and strip it of its natural oils, so then another chemical is added to make your skin softer. Maybe our ancestors had it right when they first invented the bar soap in 2800 BC and used it for face, body, hair, and clothes.

Like your skin care products, shampoos, shower gels, and hand soaps are filled with preservatives because they have a high content of water. They wash off, so there is less of a chance to absorb into the skin (although I am sure some probably does, however small). The concern here is allergens and harshness of "soaps." Allergies can some-times be severe, or in my case, a constant itchy scalp and skin. Many times I have thought my grade schooler brought home lice, and it was the shampoo ingredients. And surprise! Many people lie about what's in the product. In most cases, the "natural" companies are the worst offenders because it is difficult to create a shampoo that is all natural and won't make your hair feel like steel wool (particularly if it is color treated or highlighted).

COMMON SOAP BASES

Soap bases are usually the second ingredient, right after water. All are derived from highly processed oils of coconut, palm, or sugar, and you won't know which unless they state it on the label. This is an issue if you are allergic to one of them or if you have concerns about the over use of palm oil, which is a definite environmental concern.[1] The demand for coconut oil has grown tremendously, too, and it is not without its concerns—primarily labor abuse and farmers being taken advantage of in pricing. To avoid this, look for labels that have organic and fair trade seals, which mean the farmers were paid more and that they practice sustainable farming.

Sodium Laurel Sulfate (SLS)

Impact on Your Health

This will be a shocker if you remember the Internet scare awhile back on this ingredient, but SLS does not cause cancer or have carcinogens in it (that goes to its relative sodium *laureth* sulfate). Sodium *lauryl* sulfate is not ethoxylated like nearly every other soap. It is the ethoxylation process where contamination with 1.4 dioxane occurs. A tank that is not cleaned properly could also cross-contaminate, particularly because most of these soap bases can be made in the same facility. SLS can be derived from coconut oil through processing (like Velveeta™ cheese is derived from milk), and it can also be derived from petroleum oil. There is no way to tell unless it is declared in the label's ingredient listing. Because SLS has been around for years, it has a lot of data and research, which is good. Explore the following URL to get the full picture, https://www.ncbi.nlm.nih.gov/pmc/articles/PMC4651417/.

The concern with SLS is that it is harsh and an irritant. It cleans well and is good in laundry but not so great for your hair. In fact, it can strip your clothes of their colors, so imagine what it will do to your new high-lights. If you have sensitive skin or hair color you want to keep looking bright, SLS is not something you want to use in your shampoo or shower gel. However, it is not the carcinogen it has been made out to be and is better than its counterparts. I would use it over sodium laureth sulfate, which I will cover next. But I would not use it on a baby or child because it is too harsh for their young skin.

Impact on the Environment

In its undiluted form, SLS has moderate toxicity to fish. All SLS is diluted in products, but this world uses a lot, so what about accumulation over time? According to the thorough study found in the journal *Ecotoxicology and Environmental Safety*, the answer is no, it does not have accumulation risks but that is largely dependent on the water hardness, the species, and the water temperature.[2] It does go on to say that plant-derived substances (coconut or palm oil) are preferred because they completely biodegrade and the petroleum derived SLS does not—only 76 percent of it does and it leaves behind petroleum derivatives in the water.

Sodium Laureth Sulfate (SLES)

Impact on Your Health

SLES was what many switched to after the Internet scare came out about SLS. It was thought to be a gentler version of SLS, but unfortunately it is ethoxylated, and therefore subject to contamination to 1,4-dioxane, which is a carcinogen. SLES is also found in your shampoos and shower gels and can also be called sodium dodecyl sulfate or sodium lauryl ether sulfate.

Impact on the Environment

The biodegradability is less than 76 percent.

Cocamide MEA and DEA

Impact on Your Health

Cocamide MEA is another common surfactant found in shampoos and shower gels and foaming products. It is derived from coconut oil and can also be used as a thickener. It is relatively innocuous, and the concern is that it can sometimes be contaminated with cocamide DEA.

Cocamide DEA is a Prop 65 (a law in California requiring that a carcinogen be clearly labeled on products) chemical known to cause cancer based on the assessment done by the International Agency for Research on Cancer, which studied the exposure of the chemical on animal's skin.[3] DEA is regulated in the EU and only allowed in limited amounts and products.

Impact on the Environment

MEA is slightly toxic to aquatic life and fully biodegrades in twenty-eight days. Bioaccumulation is unknown. DEA is moderately toxic to aquatic life and also biodegrades in twenty-eight days. Bioaccumulation is unknown.

How to Detox

If bar soap is an option for you, that is the best option, both health and environmentally speaking. A good bar of soap can wash your hair, your hands, your body, your clothes—pretty much everything—and the ingredients are simple; vegetable oil (usually olive or coconut oil), water, and vitamin E or grapeseed extract. If your hair can tolerate this, it is what I recommend. You just can't get more economical or natural and you won't need preservatives. The common bars at the drugstore are not natural, so don't be fooled. Read your labels and look for minimal ingredients. Soap is simple so the ingredients will be in words you can understand. If they are not, avoid them.

If you have color-treated or highlighted hair, and you need something that is gentle here are some suggestions that are chemicals but are derived from coconut, palm, or sugar:

- Lauryl Glucoside
- Coco-Betaine or Cocomidopropyl Betaine
- Sodium Cocoyl Glutamate
- Decyl Glucoside

There are few chemical-free options in the liquid soap category. Castile soap is great but has a very high pH, which can sting and irritate and also be harsh on hair. It is not recommended for processed or color-treated hair. African black soap (the actual soap, not the brand), which is made from plantain and cocoa pod ash, is another option. I have tried soap nuts in many products and have not found them to be effective at cleaning anything.

Petroleum Ingredients

Many of the ingredients, including the surfactants (soap base), can also be petroleum derived, and there is no way of telling unless the manufacturer lists it on the bottle. As I discussed previously, petroleum is an environmental concern. The drilling, refining, and burning of oil is a major contributor to climate change and the destruction of our environment, and there is no disputing this. Petroleum products are mainly used as a "fake" emollients in lieu of expensive oils. Here are more petroleum ingredients commonly found in soaps.

All PEGs

Tetrasodium or disodium EDTA is a chelator that "grabs" and "binds"; this chemical is used to remove soap scum. Propylene glycol (PPG) is used in antifreeze and also seen in skin creams. They add it to soften or to keep liquids from freezing. DMDM hydantoin is a harmful preservative that is a formaldehyde releaser. Cetereaths is an emollient to make hair and skin feel soft. Dimethicone, or any ingredient with a *Dimeth* in the beginning (e.g., dimethiconol) is in everything related to hair. It is a silicone and leaves a coating, giving the appearance of shine, softness, and manageability. Because it leaves a coating, your skin can get clogged. Whenever I use products with this I get breakouts on my neck.

Impact on Your Health

Health wise, petroleum's manufacturing process has cross-contamination concerns with 1,4-dioxane, potentially making it tainted with carcinogens. It is used because it is cheap, plentiful, and has no odor. Like our surplus of corn and soy, manufacturers will continue to process an ingredient to get as much profit out of it as they can.

Impact on the Environment

The use of petroleum-derived products will continue our dependency on oil, which is a significant contributor to greenhouse gas emissions that cause climate change.

How to Detox

Use a natural bar soap whenever possible. Use liquid Castile soaps for hand washing and shower gels. These two steps alone would minimize use of petroleum.

Synthetic Microbeads

These are the little beads suspended in shower gels, face washes, and some hand-washing products to provide a scrubbing texture. They were banned in the United States as of 2017 and will be soon in the EU and Canada, but at the time of writing they were not banned in the United Kingdom and there are no plans to do so. Many companies have voluntarily pulled the beads from their products when it was found our water systems were being polluted by them. They do not biodegrade, so fish eat them and they do not metabolize, which means you have probably eaten them too. If you see a product with suspended beads, check the label for these ingredients: polyethylene (PE), polypropylene (PP), polyethylene terephthalate (PET), polymethyl methacrylate (PMMA), polytetrafluoroethylene (PTFE), and nylon. Instead look for scrubs that use sugar, walnut shells, sand, or rice flour.

Impact on Your Health

These little beads are being ingested by fish and then by you.

Impact on the Environment

The impacts are huge. They do not biodegrade and are polluting our water every day.

How to Detox

Until they are completely off the shelves, do not buy them. If you see colored beads suspended in a product, this is most likely plastic. Read the label for the aforementioned ingredients or just skip. I know they are fun and pretty, but think of eating them in your fish, and it will definitely take away their cuteness.

Antibacterial Ingredients

Found in shampoos and hand washes, antibacterial products promise to keep you healthy when in fact they do the exact opposite. Just recently the FDA banned nineteen antibacterial chemicals because they were proven not to work and their safety was also not proven.[4] They can no longer be used in hand soaps, though oddly they can be used in other products, which makes no sense. This is what happens when you give health responsibility to the manufacturers who puts commerce over safety. The banned ingredients include the following:

- Cloflucarban
- Fluorosalan
- Hexachlorophene
- Hexylresorcinol
- Iodine complex (ammonium ether sulfate and polyoxyethylene sorbitan monolaurate)
- Iodine complex (phosphate ester of alkylaryloxy polyethylene glycol)
- Nonylphenoxypoly (ethyleneoxy) ethanoliodine
- Poloxamer-iodine complex
- Povidone-iodine 5 to 10 percent
- Undecoylium chloride iodine complex
- Methylbenzethonium chloride
- Phenol (greater than 1.5 percent)
- Phenol (less than 1.5 percent) 16
- Secondary amyltricresols
- Sodium oxychlorosene
- Tribromsalan
- Triclocarban
- Triclosan
- Triple dye

Along with hand soap, they are found in toothpaste, deodorant, shaving cream, cutting boards (to prevent germs while contaminating your food), clothing, cosmetics, and acne products.

Impact on Your Health

All should be avoided, but I want to call out Triclosan and Triclocarban in particular. Both are endocrine disruptors and have been found in breast milk and urine in large portions of the population. Recent studies have shown Triclosan causes liver damage and may develop into tumors.[5]

Impact on the Environment

Triclosan is one of the top chemicals found in streams and fresh water bodies all over the United States.

How to Detox

Warm water and pure soap are the best and healthiest way to kill germs. By using antibacterial products, you are compromising your health. If you are concerned about germs on your hands, carry natural wipes or a natural, essential oil hand sanitizer.

CONDITIONERS

Many of us need a good conditioner so we can get a comb through our hair and using just a shampoo isn't an option. Natural options can cause heaviness and weigh down hair, making fine hair look greasy after washing. This is why chemicals and petroleum products are the main ingredient in most conditioners. Silicones, like dimethicone, are not heavy and do the trick of providing manageability and shine without wearing the hair down.

Here are some common unnatural ingredients found in hair conditioners, in addition to PEGs, dimethicone, silicones, and glycols, mentioned previously in shampoos and soaps.

- Cetyl alcohol and stearyl alcohol: These are not alcohols in the sense you know alcohol to be. They are what is called a fatty alcohol, derived from petroleum (although can be derived from plants). They are used to make your hair feel manageable and soft.
- Cyclopentasiloxane (also called D4 and D5): This was found by the EU to be an endocrine disrupter. OEHHA has concerns that it bio

accumulates and increases uterine tumors in animals. It is harmful to the environment and is found in our freshwater sources.[6]

- Behentrimonium chloride, also known as docosyltrimethylammonium chloride or BTAC-228: This is an irritant, toxic, and slightly flammable. It is used as an antistatic agent and a disinfectant. It is commonly found in cosmetics such as conditioners, hair dye, mousse, and also in detergents. In water treatment, it acts as an algaecide. So you can put it on your hair and in your pool.

Impact on Your Health

It varies on the ingredient. I am comfortable with a little dimethicone and the cetyl/stearyl alcohols and would use them during the day, but not at night because it gives me neck acne. I avoid all those that are endocrine disrupters.

How to Detox

Finding the right natural conditioner will be a matter of trial and error. There are many brands out there, but it will depend on your hair type.

Here are products I have tried and enjoyed:

- Andalou Naturals[7]
- Avalon Organics[8]
- Juice Organics[9]

CHAPTER 3

BEAUTY PRODUCTS

I KIND OF LAUGH at all the years I spent wearing (and the thousands of dollars I spent on buying) makeup, nail polish, and perfume, with no idea what was in it. Like most I was drawn to the pretty colors and transformation that they promised; health and safety was the last thing on my mind. I just assumed they were fine.

For something we put on our skin every day, and leave on for eight hours or more, we should really take a close look at the ingredients and at least know what we are putting on our skin. There are some good choices out there now, and the more we can spread the word on healthier choices the better.

In my twenties and thirties, I wore more makeup than I do now in my late forties. If this is the case for you too, please share this chapter with the young girls in your life, who are growing up and being exposed to this powerful industry. I also highly recommend you read the full studies by the FDA on cosmetics and heavy metals.[1]

MAKEUP, FRAGRANCES, AND NAIL POLISH

Eyeshadows, Blushes, and Face Powders

These three powder products contain mostly the same ingredients. A base (powder or cream), colorant, and preservatives. The size and density of the pigment are the main difference. Cream bases are also similar in all three products as well. First let's look at the powders.

Talc

Talc is the primary ingredient in most powder eyeshadows, blushes, and face powders—loose or pressed—and is usually the first ingredient. Talc is a clay mineral that is mined, and where talc grows, so does tremolite, a form of amphibole asbestos. Both come from magnesium silicate so to find them next to one another is quite common; asbestos can run through the talc like a vein. It is commonly used in baby powders, body powders, face powders, eye shadows, bronzers, and blushes.

Impact on Your Health

Talc has been monitored since the 1970s for asbestos contamination and the FDA says commercial talc used in beauty and hygiene products should be asbestos free. Although talc is checked for asbestos, contamination can still happen as a result of poor mining practices. Not every batch of talc mined is monitored, and when it is sourced from countries with less regulations, contamination can occur. Another concern with talc is tumor growth. A study in 1993 on rats found that talc causes tumors on its own—with or without asbestos contamination. This U.S. National Toxicology Program report found that cosmetic-grade talc containing no asbestos-like fibers was correlated with tumor formation in rats forced to inhale talc for 6 hours a day, 5 days a week over at least 113 weeks.[2] Granted that is a lot of talc to inhale, however something to think about if you use a lot of loose powder. Overall inhalation of talc is something you need to avoid because the tiny particles adhere to your lungs. Every time you powder your face or body, you are inhaling it. There is a protocol from OSHA for any worker who works with soapstone/talc, and they must be protected from dust.

I realize no one is blasting talc mines in their beauty routine; however I wouldn't use it in a loose powder and certainly not around infants or children. I remember playing with baby powder as a kid and making dust storms in the air. Not even guessing this was damaging to my lungs. In 2016, a large lawsuit was settled by Johnson and Johnson for millions of dollars to the plaintiff's surviving family who blamed Johnson and Johnson's body powder for her death from ovarian cancer.[3] She used the powder in her underwear daily to stay fresh as recommended. The daily use of talc was pinpointed to be the cause of her tumor growth in her ovaries. There are thousands more such cases awaiting trial.

Contamination is less of a concern but also an unknown. Thousands of tons of talc are mined, and they are not all checked for asbestos. There are no guarantees the talc used is asbestos free. I think this is an ingredient you can easily avoid and should be cautious with. Cornstarch and rice powder are good replacements.

Impact on the Environment

Talc is a natural resource that is mined all around the world. It is depleted in India, but people still illegally mine—often in untouched land such as protected nature preserves. This not only harms the environment, but also the endangered animals who live there. The mining of talc is not sustainable and will eventually run out. Lastly, the talc mining industry also supports the practice of hiring persons who are not protected by unions and made to work under dangerous conditions.

How to Detox

There are many alternatives to talc powder. Mineral makeup, rice powder, and cornstarch are just a few. Mineral-based makeup uses safer minerals, but they are still being mined. The colorants are also food-grade coloring and can be derived from animal sources (see next topic). I prefer a rice powder- or cornstarch-based makeup. Many brands have made the switch from talc, and it should be easy to find at your local beauty counter.

Cream Eyeshadows, Blushes, and Makeup

These are usually better to use—just make sure they are free of acrylates such as methacrylate, which has toxic concerns.[4] You will also find silicones in many of them, such as dimethicone, which is also used to make your hair soft and shiny. It makes my skin breakout, so I avoid it on my skin. Look for a natural brand that uses oils such as coconut oil and beeswax instead.

Colorants

Colors and dyes in makeup (and food) are something I try to avoid, but they are unavoidable in makeup. Many come from natural sources, and before the 1900s, natural ingredients were used all the time. They also contained mercury, copper, and arsenic. Our Earth's soil and crust contains many things, including trace amounts of heavy metals, and in some cases, poison. Today the dyes we use are almost exclusively made from coal tar/petroleum. Colorants with FD&C or D&C in the name are synthetic or derived from coal tar. D&C means they are approved just for drugs and cosmetics; FD&C includes food approval.

A "Lake" is a mixture of a dye or FD&C colorant with a pure colorant (not water soluble) and aluminum salts to create a new color. Lake plus aluminum salt plus FD&C Blue No.1 would be FD&C Blue No. 1, Aluminum Lake.[5] The numbers indicate the version of the color created. Lakes can also be natural and come from sources such as beets, achiote seeds, turmeric, and others.

Some natural colorants such as mineral makeup have their issues too. Iron oxides—titanium dioxide, zinc oxide, and micas—are all natural minerals, but still cosmetic companies will combine them with synthetic pigments to get the color they want. Mineral makeup is limited to "earth tones," which makes sense because it is coming from the earth. If you see a bright color—blue, purple, green—this is a good sign it is mixed. Although minerals are natural, just like talc, they are fine, and the small particles are being inhaled. Something to think about if you use large amounts.

Lastly some natural colorants come from insects, and if you are a vegan, you may not even know you are wearing bugs. Cochineal or carmine (also known as carminic acid) are derived from the crushed carcasses of a South and Central American female insect called *Dactylopius coccus*.

Impact on Your Health

The concern is in the quality of the colorant. If it were as simple as buying it from a few people, the ingredients could be monitored. However, this is not the case. Colorants come from all over the world, and heavy metal contamination occurs all the time. As recently as 2016, Halloween makeup was recalled for high content of heavy metals, including lead.[6] Although the initial colorant is tested for approval, the process thereafter is not. The FDA requires some colors to be tested with every single batch (presumably because the risk of contamination is particularly high with those colors) but not all. So once a color is approved, it is assumed that everyone is getting good quality ingredients. I am not comfortable with assumptions. Natural minerals pose a risk because they are often mixed with synthetics. Natural minerals also can be contaminated with heavy metals. And like talc, the super fine particles are a health concern when inhaled and can cause lung damage if inhaled over time in significant amounts.

Carmine or the "bug dye" has caused allergic reactions. A request to the FDA to warn consumers of this potential allergic reaction was denied. Instead of listing the ingredient as an insect, it will continue to list it by carmine or cochineal extract. If you are a vegetarian or unaware of what those words mean, you are unknowingly wearing or ingesting something you don't want to, which doesn't seem fair. Other than allergies, no other health affects have been discovered to my knowledge.

Social and Environmental Impact

Natural minerals such as mica are mined and 60 percent of mica is mined in India. India has a huge child labor issue, and 86 percent of the mica exports were unregulated. Mica purchasing is also increasing every year because of consumer desires for a more "natural" product. If it doesn't come from India, then it could come from China or Africa—other countries who have also failed to ban child labor. It is not sustainable and once it is all mined, it is gone. Carmine or cochineal insects are farmed, and Peru is the largest importer.

How to Detox

There are several makeup lines emerging who use natural fruit and spice pigments. Although the palette is limited, this is a good option for those concerned (see Resources chapter).

Lipstick

Considering we put this on our mouths daily and eat about one and a half pounds over a lifetime, it is worthy of examination. The FDA has guidelines and approves the colorants, but the ingredients are sourced and monitored by the company who makes them. If no one tests, anything could be in there. The bases of lipstick are made up of many waxes and oil—natural ones too—and then various ingredients such as polyethylene (which is a plastic), preservatives, and fragrance are added.

Like eyeshadows, blushes, and face powders, lipstick colorants also have the potential for contamination. In 2007 the Campaign for Safe Cosmetics found lead to be in high amounts in the lipsticks they tested. They informed the FDA, and three years later, the FDA

Table 3.1

Sample Number	Brand	Parent Company	Lipstick Line Shade Number Shade	Lot Number[a]	Lead (Pb)[b] (ppm)
1	Maybelline	L'Oréal USA	Color Sensational 125 Pink Petal	FF205	7.19
2	L'Oréal	L'Oréal USA	Colour Riche 410 Volcanic	FE259	7.00
3	NARS	Shiseido	Semi-Matte 1005 Red Lizard	OKAW	4.93
4	Cover Girl Queen Collection	Procter & Gamble	Vibrant Hues Color Q580 Ruby Remix	9139	4.92

[a] Lot numbers embossed or printed on lipstick cases or end labels.
[b] Results are for total lead content determined by FDA's validated method.
Source: http://www.fda.gov/cosmetics/productsingredients/products/ucm137224.htm#initial _survey.

published their own findings. The FDA recommends no more than 10 ppm, but as you can see, the lead content was as high as 7.19 ppm. (The full study can be found in Table 3.1.)

Impact on Your Health

If you wear lipstick every day like me, it is worth your while to use one that has a natural base. Department store brands commonly use castor oil and candelilla wax, along with plastics, silicones, preservatives, and fragrances. The preservatives you find in your shampoo are also in lipsticks. Anything with colorants (e.g., D&C, FD&C, Lake, or color with a number after it) along with mica and oxides, all have the potential to have heavy metals in them. Heavy metals are something we are exposed to every day; it is in our water and the food we eat because it is naturally in our soil and in air pollution, leaving its residue on anything grown outdoors. For perspective, see the following studies showing the heavy metal content found in fruits and vegetables: "Analysis of Mineral and Heavy Metal Content of Some Commercial Fruit Juices by Inductively Coupled Plasma Mass Spectrometry"[7] and "Determination of Heavy Metals in the Fruit of Date Palm Growing at Different Locations of Riyadh."[8] Lipstick heavy metal exposure is there, but probably minimal next to the foods and juices we drink.

Impact on the Environment

Besides packaging and the inclusion of minerals (see Colorants section), the impact is minimal.

How to Detox

Use a brand that has a natural base such as beeswax and oils you can recognize (e.g., coconut, jojoba). Natural fruit dyes and the FD&C colorants all have some sort of heavy metal content, but if made in the United States, it should be minimal. I would avoid any lipstick made in China because they have been shown to have much higher contents of heavy metals in their products.

Mascara

In 1933 a product called Lash Lure, an eyelash dye using a toxic coal tar colorant called paraphenylenediamine, caused blindness in thirteen women. It took the bravery of Ruth de Forest Lamb and her book, *American Chamber of Horrors*, about the FDA's lack of policing consumer products to bring much needed awareness. Today we have come a long way, but we should always be careful when we put anything next to our eyes.

Impact on Your Health

Most mascara concerns are with allergies and irritation. Usually preservatives and colorants and sometimes perfumes are to blame. A mascara can contain twenty-five ingredients or more, making it difficult to pinpoint what may be irritating our eyes. Colorants such as carmine (the insects) and ingredients such as talc can also be in there.

Impact on the Environment

Besides packaging and the inclusion of minerals (see Colorants section), the impact is minimal.

How to Detox

Look for mascaras without fragrance, talc, and harmful colorants. Natural mascaras have not quite caught up performance wise, and you will most likely try several before you find the right one. Physicians Formula has several natural options and are widely available at chain drugstores, many of which have good return policies on makeup. So you can experiment knowing you can return them if it doesn't work out. Mascaras will always have a preservative and should. The act of taking the wand in and out and exposing it to your lashes and air and reusing it several times makes this product extremely prone to bacteria. To not use a preservative would be careless.

Fragrances

Scent is the number-one memory inducing sense we have. The experience of smelling something and being transported to an event or place is something that has happened to all of us. It can have a pleasurable effect (pumpkin spice) or an unpleasant one (the smell of gin after drinking too much of it). Nearly everything we use has a fragrance in it. Shampoos, toothpaste, detergent, air spray, car fresheners, even clothing stores and hotels have signature fragrances associated with them. Considering you can remember someone by the scent of their shampoo; it is a powerful marketing tool.

Fragrances are created using synthetic, petroleum-based ingredients and natural essences/oils. Synthetic ingredients are usually a 50:50 mix of petroleum and naturals. The use of synthetic oils allows for perfumes to be stronger and smell more like the "real" scent. A garden rose smells nothing like the scent of its essential oil, rose otto. The essential oil has a much earthier profile, is more than $1,000 an ounce, and fades within an hour or two of wearing it. The use of synthetic ingredients allows for a scent that smells exactly like the rose you sniffed in your garden and will last long.

On the other side of the coin are natural fragrances, which are derived from many sources. They can come from fruits, flowers, and in the case of musk such as civet, animals (although this is not practiced by most anymore and a synthetic is used).

Perfume companies generally do not share their ingredients—even with the companies buying them. It is considered top secret, and they have the right to not disclose it. But all this secrecy is not working to anyone's benefit and is creating more skepticism of the industry.

The perfume industry has two trade organizations that independently monitor the chemicals used—including natural ones too—in the industry for safety on a regular basis. Their names are RIFM and IFRA. They provide perfumers with updated safety information, as well as recommended percentages.

When a manufacturer purchases a perfume, they can make sure it is from a company that follows the guidelines set out by these organizations, which is there to ensure safety. I would add they are probably ahead of the FDA on many ingredients and work faster, as they are nongovernmental entities. They are also supported by the perfumers who created it. Some may say this is not a truly "independent" organization then.

In my discussions with experts on this topic on both the natural and synthetic side, most agreed that the perfume industry would not consciously use bad ingredients. But how can you tell what is good and what is bad on the shelf? You can't.

And natural doesn't mean carcinogen free; there are many essential oils out there, which are 100% natural, but contain carcinogens, mutagens, and reproductive disruptors. In fact, you are exposed to carcinogens all the time when you eat and drink—and not by a manufacturer's hand, but Mother Nature's. When you eat basil or drink your warm lemon juice in the morning, you are also ingesting acetaldehyde, a natural by-product of oxidation and a known human carcinogen. It is found in many foods known to also have anticancer effects, such as broccoli, apples, onions, oranges, strawberries, lemons, and mushrooms. It should also be noted that there is no difference in harm if the carcinogen is in its natural form or a synthetic match.

Lastly, preservatives are often hidden in a fragrance. They can be a sneaky way for natural companies to say they are "preservative free" because it is hidden in the fragrance and doesn't need to be listed. Some preservatives can also be a scent ingredient. One preservative, phenoxyethanol, is used for aroma purposes. The company using the fragrance in their product may not even know. There are many reasons, but for those with preservative allergies, it can be a game of Russian roulette.

Impact on Your Health

Fragrances have possible contamination with preservatives and chemicals that are harmful to the endocrine system and are potential carcinogens and mutagens. A potential allergic reaction in the form of rashes, hives, and itchiness is also a concern.

Impact on the Environment

There is no way of knowing if any synthetic fragrance is biodegradable because we don't know the ingredients. Many ingredients—also found in fragrance—are also found in our fresh water. This is no surprise, given everything from your hand soap to your shower gel to your unfragranced laundry detergent has fragrance in it.

Natural fragrances and oils biodegrade.

How to Detox

If you want to be absolutely free of carcinogens, endocrine disruptors, and mutagens in your fragrance, you will have to do research on the essential oils and their constituents. Essential oil expert and well-respected teacher Robert Tisserand has a book titled "*Essential Oil Safety*." You can find all you need to know on essential oils there.

A synthetic fragrance will be far more difficult because you will not know the ingredients to begin with, unless they are all disclosed.

I think moderation is key. If you enjoy a fragrance, wear it but maybe don't spray as much. I enjoy fragrance but I no longer wear a perfume daily. Oddly I get many more compliments now on how good I smell. Go figure.

Nail Polish

When you open a bottle, it should be clear that nail polish is not natural in any shape or form. If you do a Google search on natural nail polishes, many articles and products come up. But the fact is they all contain ingredients that may be formaldehyde free but are hardly natural, and I would say it is a stretch to also call them toxic free. To make the shiny, chip-free colors, they have to use ingredients that are essentially liquid plastic. Daily use of nail polish makes your nails brittle, flaky, and damaged. When you use polish, you are literally stopping your nails from breathing. The fumes aren't great either. A 2002 study (Table 3.2) determined that the constant inhalation of fumes by nail technicians did indeed slow them down cognitively.[9]

Impact on Your Health

Many of the ingredients found in nail polishes are also carcinogens. Use polishes that are free of formaldehyde, toluene, DBP, camphor, parabens, and TBHP. The colorants are all derived from coal tar, so even if you took out all the plasticizers and carcinogens, you still would have something harmful that is on your skin—all the time. There is a company that makes polish for kids that is water based, using acetate copolymer as an adhesive and colorants that are again FD&C colorants, derived from coal tar. The water base is much better and will also be close to fume free. I have no idea if it provides the "look" of a clean polished nail because I have not used it.

Impact on the Environment

Nail polish is not biodegradable.

How to Detox

After religiously getting my nails done every week, I stopped all polish and do not recommend it. A buffed nail will give a beautiful shine and

Table 3.2

Acetone Material Safety Data Sheet (MSDS)	
IV. Fire and Explosion Data	
Flash Point	1.4
Flammable Limits in Air (% By Volume)	
Lower	2.5%
Upper	12.8%
Auto Ignition Temperature	869° F
Unusual Fire and Explosion Hazards	Use water spray. Use water spray to cool fire exposed tanks and containers. Acetone/water solutions that contain more than 2.5% acetone have flash points. When the acetone concentration is greater than 8% (by weight) in a closed container, it would be within flammable range and cause fire or explosion if a source of ignition were introduced.
Fire-Extinguishing Media	Water spray, alcohol resistant foam, dry chemical, or carbon dioxide.

SOURCE: http://mfc.engr.arizona.edu/safety/MSDS%20FOLDER/Acetone.pdf

will look healthy because it is healthy. My nails are stronger than they have ever been. I would never use polish on a child's nails, and if it is used, I would remove it in twenty-four hours.

Nail Polish Remover

I don't need to tell you this is toxic, you just need to open a bottle and smell it. They all contain some form of a solvent because they are used to remove paint—just not on the walls but your fingers and toes.

Impact on Your Health

Most store brands use acetone. Here are the harms of acetone straight from its MSDS.

It causes dermatitis and has potential nervous system effects such as headaches, nausea, and dizziness and is fatal if swallowed (see Table 3.2).

Impact on the Environment

It is a hazardous substance and cannot be poured down the drain, although I am pretty sure thousands do.

How to Detox

Use a remover that is acetone free and uses safer ingredients such as propylene carbonate or ethyl acetate and isopropyl alcohol. It should be noted that even if it is found in Whole Foods or in a "natural" store, remover is not a natural product. It is a solvent—even if some of the ingredients included are natural. These are added for skin softening because the solvent will dry your skin—and also for marketing, so you feel better about applying a solvent to your skin.

CHAPTER 4

DENTAL HYGIENE

A BRIGHT, WHITE smile is the ultimate in good dental health, right? This is what we are told and this is also what we are sold. In the United States alone, oral care products are near 1 billion in revenue. But how safe are all these products we use to have cleaner, whiter teeth? Are they helpful or just another story we have been told by marketers and advertisers? This chapter will take a look at these important products we use daily and the safety of the ingredients in them.

TOOTHPASTE

Brushing our teeth twice a day, every day is a no brainer. As soon as we have teeth, we are taught the importance of taking care of them and our gums. The fear of cavities is real and what parent hasn't scolded their child for not brushing well enough after a bad trip to the dentist? Toothpaste alone is a $12.6 billion dollar industry—that is more than some countries's annual gross domestic product (GDP).[1]

I personally have not used a "regular" toothpaste since 2014, nor has my son. I wish someone had told me how unhealthy the ingredients in toothpaste were years ago, but like me, they probably never dreamed the ingredients would be unhealthy. Really who would ever think the stuff we clean our mouths with—and inevitably swallow—every day is harmful.

Here is a look at the ingredients found in all big brand toothpastes and some—like carrageenan—are also in natural products.

- Colgate Total Advanced Whitening Toothpaste—Active Ingredients: Sodium fluoride 0.24% (0.15% w/v fluoride ion)—Anticavity, Triclosan 0.30%—Antigingivitis—Inactive Ingredients: water, hydrated silica, glycerin, sorbitol, PVM/MA copolymer, sodium lauryl sulfate, flavor, cellulose gum, sodium hydroxide, propylene glycol, carrageenan, sodium saccharin, titanium dioxide.
- Aquafresh Extreme Clean—Active Ingredient: sodium fluoride 0.25% (0.15% w/v fluoride ion) Inactive Ingredients: water, hydrated silica, sorbitol, glycerin, PEG-8, sodium lauryl sulfate, flavor, anthan gum, titanium dioxide, cocamidopropyl betaine, sodium saccharin, iron oxide, red 30.
- Crest Pro-Health Whitening Power—Active Ingredient: stannous fluoride 0.454% (0.14% w/v fluoride ion)—Inactive Ingredients: water, sorbitol, hydrated silica, sodium lauryl sulfate, carrageenan, sodium gluconate, flavor, xanthan gum, zinc citrate, stannous chloride, sodium hydroxide, sodium saccharin, sucralose, mica, titanium dioxide, Blue 1.

I examined the ingredients of these brand-name whitening toothpastes, although you will find most of these ingredients in all drugstore toothpastes.

Sodium Hexametaphosphate

Sodium hexametaphosphate is an inorganic phosphate salt added to toothpaste for antistaining and tartar buildup. It is also a food additive. In this medical study, rats who were fed a 10 percent solution of sodium hexametaphosphate had pale and swollen kidneys.[2]

Sorbitol

Sorbitol is usually derived from corn oil and is a sugar substitute because toothpaste manufacturers aren't going to use real sugar so a synthetic one is used. Sorbitol is added to "sweeten" the toothpaste, make it more palatable, and give it a transparent look. Sorbitol has been shown to cause gastrointestinal upset and is used also as a laxative.

Sodium Lauryl Sulfate

Sodium lauryl sulfate is a strong detergent that is used in everything from floor soap to laundry detergent. It is omitted from many shampoos because it can strip color. In toothpaste, there are many reports it causes canker sores. This is added to give toothpaste a foaming characteristic.

Propylene Glycol

Propylene glycol is a petroleum product added to bring moisture to your mouth, probably because of the drying caused by the sodium lauryl sulfate. It can also be derived from glycerin, which can come from animal fat, vegetable fat, or petroleum. It is found in antifreeze and skin creams as well. It can be an allergen for some people; if you experience redness around the mouth, this could be from the propylene glycol in your toothpaste.

Carrageenan

Carrageenan is naturally derived from red seaweed. It sounds innocuous; however it has been shown to cause gastrointestinal problems, including causing a higher risk of ulcerations and intestinal inflammation. Because it is derived from natural sources, it is used in many "health" products as a thickener, including soy, almond, and coconut milks.[3]

For those with irritable bowel syndrome or Crohn's disease, this ingredient can be a big issue.

Fluoride

There are many opposing studies on fluoride. Some feel that tooth decay prevention trumps any reports that fluoride is also a neurotoxin and causes a decline in IQ. Others feel that fluoride was approved far too quickly without enough testing.

Regardless, the facts show that the rise of fluorosis (too much fluoride) has increased.[4] My son has yellowing of the teeth from too much fluoride. Unfortunately, I was not aware of this until most of his adult teeth came in. He now uses a nonfluoride toothpaste. Fluoride is a naturally occurring substance in our water and its levels can be high. It was first discovered in 1909 when the residents of a small town in Colorado were finding mysterious dark brown spots on their teeth. After many years of investigation, it was found that the town's drinking water (which came from local springs) had too much fluoride. The residents were suffering from fluorosis. In turn, they also found that the brown spots were preventing decay. So, in 1945, fluoride was added nationwide to public drinking water. After eleven years it was found the cavity rate declined in

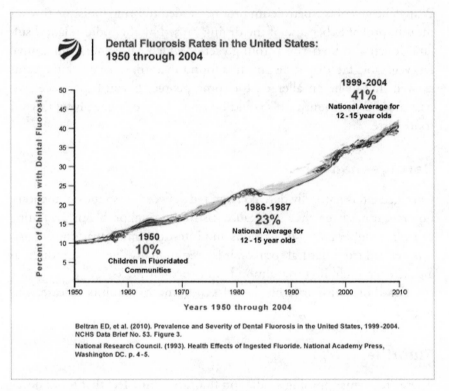

Figure 4.1
Source: World Health Organization

the children by 60 percent. This was proof enough and now more than 70 percent of states in the United States have fluoride added to their water.

Fast forward seventy years later, *Newsweek* published an article stating that there are few studies (since the adding of fluoride to water) to show that fluoride deters cavities and decay.[5]

Fluoride may or may not prevent tooth decay, but its use over time is detrimental to our health and right now we have poor monitoring of the amount we are taking in. It is in our water, our toothpaste, and our mouthwashes.

Too much fluoride is a neurotoxin and can cause lowering of IQ, joint pain, and thyroid issues. We know that fluorosis is way up and the U.S. Department of Health and Human Services agrees because it just reduced the fluoride levels added to water because of this dramatic increase—which should have been done years ago when we started adding it to our toothpastes as well. Many dentists blame the overuse of amoxicillin for mottling teeth because overuse of fluoride is something that most dentists do not want to acknowledge.

Colorants

Colorants are in your toothpaste and sadly are most prevalent in children's brands. They include mica, titanium dioxide, and the coal tar derived Blue 1. As discussed in previous chapters, colorants can often be contaminated with heavy metals and arsenic.

Xylitol

This is a sugar alcohol and a natural sweetener that is derived from birch wood. There have been studies showing it reduces cavities and promotes remineralization; it is also the same ingredient that is harmful to dogs. There is not enough information yet to decide on this. You will find it in many natural dental products, as well as gum and some drugstore-brand dental products. An article in *Crunchy Betty* about xylitol is worth reading, too.[6]

Triclosan

Triclosan was just removed from hand sanitizers because of concerns of ineffectiveness and being an endocrine disruptor. It is still allowed in several other products, including toothpaste.[7]

Impact on Health

Sadly, it appears that most toothpastes have a lot of ingredients to make brushing more enjoyable, but with little health benefits. In fact, we are receiving too much fluoride and some of the ingredients can cause stomach issues. Most of the ingredients are not for the health of your teeth; they are just there to bind other ingredients, make it taste better, and look cool.

Impact on the Environment

Fluoride can inhibit and increase algae, depending on concentrations, and can adversely affect invertebrates and fish.[8] Because it is added to our water, there really isn't much escaping it. I did not find concerns with the other ingredients. Triclosan is in all our water, but Colgate says it biodegrades.[9]

How to Detox

Use a toothpaste without the aforementioned ingredients. Some "natural" brands use sodium lauryl sulfate and fluoride. You must read the labels. I have recommended brands in the back of the book, but please do not assume if it is at Whole Foods it is free of these ingredients. If you are bottle-feeding your baby, do not use tap water, which is overfluorinated. Consider using a nonfluoridated toothpaste for those of toothbrushing age.

MOUTHWASHES

Mouthwashes are a marketing tool to make you think you are getting your teeth cleaner. In fact, you are rinsing with the same ingredients found in your toothpaste. In the case of Listerine®, they use the natural powers of essential oil of thyme, menthol, and eucalyptus, but then add alcohol, artificial sweeteners, colorants, and preservatives. Another ingredient, cetylpyridinium chloride, is found in other brands, which is a chemical bacterial killer.

The essential oils used in Listerine were found to be equally effective in killing germs as the chemical cetylpyridinium chloride.[10] Using some of these mouthwashes will take away your natural pH and is also like swishing your mouth with toxins. Here are some of the additional ingredients that may pose potential harm.

- Tetrapotassium pyrophosphate—This is used in laundry detergents, mouthwashes, and automotive products. It is a serious skin irritant and toxic if swallowed and is the main ingredient in most whitening rinses. Why it's included in mouthwash is a mystery.[11]
- Hydrogen peroxide—Usually found in medicine cabinets and naturally found in your body, it is a main ingredient in most whitening rinses. It causes dry mouth.
- Phosphoric acid—This is found in Listerine HEALTHYWHITE™ mouthwash. The same stuff you pour on cement to get rid of oil stains is being put in a bottle to rinse your mouth.

Impact on Your Health

The use of mouthwashes can dry out your mouth, cause mouth irritation, and change your natural pH. If you brush and floss regularly and properly, there is no need for this.

Impact on the Environment

Many of the ingredients used, like those found in toothpaste, are harmful to aquatic life.

How to Detox

There are many all natural mouth rinses using the power of essential oils, which are just as effective at killing germs. If you are looking to get in the nooks and crannies and prevent cavities, try one that uses xylitol. (It is a natural sugar alcohol, which has been shown to decrease decay but is also known to cause stomach cramps and is a laxative.) You can also try other natural remedies such as rinsing with apple cider vinegar (which will naturally kill some bacteria) and coconut oil pulling (an Ayurvedic tradition said to promote dental health and remove toxins).

WHITENERS

Most tooth whiteners use hydrogen peroxide as a whitener. The effects are temporary, but your mouth and gums can suffer. Hydrogen peroxide burns skin, so if you are a frequent user of the strips and gels, the redness, burning, and increase in sensitivity is something you may have experienced.

Impact on Your Health

Whiteners can cause mouth sores, sensitive teeth, and inflamed gums.

Impact on the Environment

The impact is negligible other than the waste of products.

How to Detox

Make your own natural whitener. Coconut oil pulling, brushing with baking soda and lemon juice, brushing with turmeric (see a blog post from mommypotamus) and activated charcoal (the kind at a health food store, not your BBQ) have all been shown to give good results and increase gum health—not harm it.[12]

DENTAL FLOSS

Most dental floss is made from nylon (which does not biodegrade and is also harmful to birds and our aquatic life where our garbage gets dumped) and it is coated with either a petroleum wax or worse, Teflon™.

Impact on Your Health

If you use the same Oral-B® floss I did, it is coated with PTFE, and as they say on their website "Polytetrafluorethylene floss (PTFE) is the same material used in high-tech Gore-Tex fabric. The material slides between the teeth easily and is less likely to shred compared to standard floss."13 It is also the same material used to make Teflon pans. PTFE is a concern, and there is no need to use it in an oral product when there are many other options.[14]

Impact on Your Health

Flossing with PTFE has health concerns because they do not break down in our body.

Impact on the Environment

Nylon floss does not biodegrade and is harmful to the birds who pick at it and drop it in our waters, which then harm our aquatic life.

How to Detox

Use a natural floss made from silk thread, which biodegrades. Natural coatings such as beeswax are best and are not harmful to your health.

PART II

DETOX YOUR KITCHEN AND PANTRY

How the Industrialization of Our Food Is Harming Us

THIS ISN'T about weight or the latest juice cleanse. This chapter is about foods that bring health and wellness to your body. In this section, we will explore that it is not just what you eat, but also how it is grown and raised that is equally as important.

After having breast cancer, food became a way to bring health into my life. I always ate well and figured organic was enough, but after reading the book, *We the Eaters*, by Ellen Gustafson, my eyes were opened to many facts, the most important one being that our health started to deteriorate when the industrialization of our food started. Gustafson is a remarkable young woman who has spent considerable time investigating food systems. Along with Lauren Bush, she co-founded FEED and worked at the UN Food Program and the Council on Foreign relations. Her resume is impressive to say the least, and she isn't even forty yet.

Gustafson sees both sides of the coin. She loves food and a good barbeque. She grew up in Pennsylvania and understands farming. She also understands poverty and malnutrition from her numerous trips for FEED and hands-on work in Africa. What Gustafson brings to the table, literally and figuratively, are her Midwestern values, Columbia education, and a passion to see our food system change to a way that is healthier and sustainable.

The problem with industrialization is that it was not fully thought out; the growth in new chemicals and petroleum products are examples. It certainly has helped to create more food than ever to a growing population, but that growth has not been managed well. For instance, you may know corn syrup isn't good for you, but do you know exactly why? Corn syrup was first invented in 1864 by the Clinton Corn Processing Company in Clinton, Iowa. It was not stable and it wasn't until 1965 to 1970, when a Japanese chemist, Yoshiyuki Takasaki, developed a heat stable enzyme, which then was licensed by Clinton Corn, and high fructose corn syrup (HFCS) became a "thing." In 1976, corn syrup began to replace sucrose as the main sweetener of soft drinks in the United States. After the introduction of corn syrup, the next three decades had a 25 percent increase in "added sugars."

And guess what also started at the exact same time? Obesity.

Corn syrup is cheap and it is also plentiful. Because of subsidies and protection by our government, we continue to grow too much corn— and not the sweet kind we can eat—but field corn, which is now feeding cows (grain), cars (ethanol), and you (corn syrup). Unfortunately, corn is not good for any of us. Cows are meant to graze and eat grass because they can't properly digest corn. When you feed a cow corn, they tend to have higher risk of infection. Ethanol derived from corn for gas is a great idea in concept; unfortunately ethanol is not as efficient as gasoline, so we use more. But to grow the corn, we need more gasoline! And for humans, corn syrup does absolutely nothing for us nutritionally or otherwise. But corn is a big business and there are billions of dollars tied in to this industry, and it will take all of us waking up and demanding that our land is used more efficiently and sustainably.

A 2016 chart (Figure P.1) shows where all the corn grown in the United States goes. This is not sweet corn, but field corn. Sweet corn is

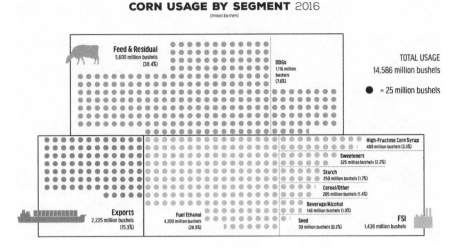

Figure P.1
Source: worldofcorn.com

nominal in production—just 2.9 billion pounds a year to regular corn, which is 150 billion pounds in the state of Iowa alone.

The good news is there are many out there fighting the good fight already. One of the "food champions" I had the pleasure of meeting is Dan Barber, author of *The Third Plate* and renowned chef of Blue Hill Farm and Blue Hill at Stone Barns. After expressing how overwhelming and daunting the situation felt, he told me to be hopeful because so much progress was being made toward eating better whole foods and that companies who stock the "center aisles" of our grocery stores, which is where the "by-products" live, are not sure where to go. The center aisle is indeed shrinking and we are making progress.

The answers are not so simple though. We are a world of billions and creating a food system that can feed everyone in health and wellness will take care, thought, flexibility, and bravery. The latter two being key—because surely there will be mistakes and something may not be the great idea it turned out to be. Bravery to put the health of billions over the wealth of thousands is where the real change will come. We can figure this out and just need to keep our moral compass pointed in the right direction.

CHAPTER 5

GMOS, ORGANIC, AND BIODYNAMIC

What Does It All Mean and Why Should I Care?

KNOWING WHAT you are eating and putting into your body is probably the single-most important thing you should care about. I find it perplexing to read posts and tweets on the horrible ingredients in shampoos, but that same person will drink a soda or eat a bag of gummy worms without thought. Part of this is possibly unawareness and a trust that our food is safe, but I think we all have been guilty of taking our bodies for granted.

My husband who hears me talk about the harms of our industrialized food supply will still buy a bag of neon orange cheese balls without even thinking. He is not alone because many of the concerns discussed in this book are not *immediately* concerning. Eating poorly will not show its ill effects until years down the road. The first sign of being overweight, and then maybe type 2 diabetes comes along. We start drugs to stop it—putting on a bandage—allowing us to continue bad habits. Before we know it, we are on insulin, blood pressure medication, cholesterol pills, and getting back surgery.

Like cosmetics, eating for your health requires some label reading on your part. Labels are deceptive—even the natural ones. Until all food companies are truly regulated and required to list how they source and grow their food, we must educate ourselves and stay aware.

If we can start educating at an early age, we can make healthy changes and food manufacturers will follow. Our body is our only car, our only house, and we can't trade it in for a new one. Once we fully understand its value, giving up the bad stuff is not only easy, but it is also a priority.

GENETICALLY MODIFIED ORGANISMS (GMOS)

GMOs are seeds whose DNA has been altered to create a new plant. Per the World Health Organization, "Genetically modified organisms (GMOs) can be defined as organisms (i.e. plants, animals or microorganisms) in which the genetic material (DNA) has been altered in a way that does not occur naturally by mating and/or natural recombination."[1]

We have long cross-bred seeds to create different and interesting foods that are also juicier and tastier. The process of creating a hybrid plant is by cross-pollination; it happens naturally and often by mistake when different crops are planted next to one another. But with GMOs, the DNA of the seed is changed and genes are spliced, which alters the DNA.

Changing a seed is not something new, and many of the foods we eat have been modified. Carrots, bananas, watermelon, and corn are all hybrids and changed from their original state. An heirloom (original) carrot is pretty much indistinguishable from our carrots today.

So why can't we just do what we are doing and cross-pollinate? Why GMOs? That is a good question. The genetically engineered seeds are being altered mainly to resist drought and the need for pesticides. Big businesses see climate change for the real problem it is, but instead of fixing it and altering their business practices, they work on new products to fill the need that will come, like drought-resistant seeds.

The idea of using less pesticide is appealing. However, opponents of GMOs would argue that pesticide use has increased because nature develops a resistance to the pesticide, and bugs, such as rootworm, modify their genetic makeup naturally to continue to feed on the pest-resistant corn and thereby creating a "super bug."[2] And that super bug that will require even more pesticide to kill it or possibly ruin an entire crop if there's not a new super bug pesticide in place. None of this takes into account the health effects of massive amounts of pesticide on our food.

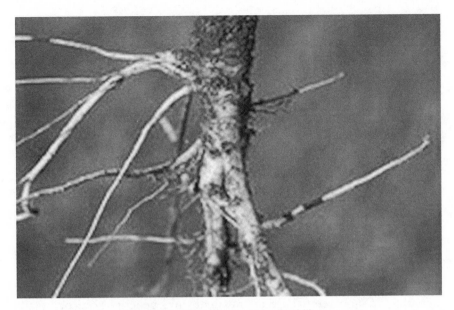

Figure 5.1 What a carrot looked like . . .
Source: GENETIC LITERACY PROJECT

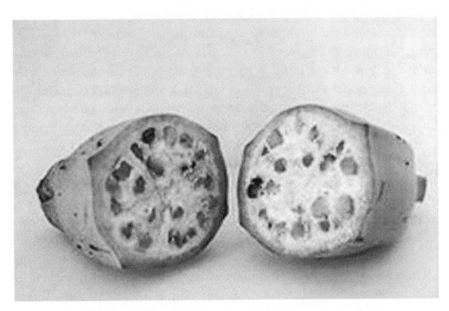

Figure 5.2 . . . and a banana.
Source: GENETIC LITERACY PROJECT

Understandably there is a desire and campaign to make it a law in the United States that GMOs be labeled. (It is already heavily regulated in the EU and banned in some places.[3])

But it is not that simple. When crops sit next to one another—say an organic broccoli and a GMO broccoli—the wind, the bees, and the pollinators naturally cross over. Now you have organic broccoli that is mixed with a GMO seed. If this continues, eventually you could just have GMO broccoli because the organic is now completely polluted.

Another concern or unknown with GMOs is nutrition and variety. Before industrialization, we used to eat many different varieties of one fruit or vegetable. A great example of this is heirloom tomatoes. Some are big, small, green, yellow—even purple. But then people started buying only the prettier ones and the others went unpurchased. Growers saw this and weeded their crops down to using only the seeds from the prettier plants. Eventually the others are nonexistent, but by removing these varieties, we also removed their nutrients and benefits from our plate. Many countries who had unique, indigenous vegetables have lost them, including the United States. In 1903 there were three hundred different varieties of corn; by 1983, we had just twelve.

Like most things right now, there is a monopoly of four to five businesses who you can get things from and the seed industry is no exception. Currently Monsanto (just purchased by Bayer Pharmaceuticals) is the only producer of GMO seed and also the manufacturer of the top-selling pesticide, Roundup (glyphosate), in the world. Having the seed seller also as the manufacturer of the pesticide is not good one-stop shopping. If they want to sell both products, why would they create a seed that uses *less* pesticide? They don't. They create a seed that will be resistant and then need a new pesticide. Or more of the other. It is a classic example of allowing too much control in the hands of too few. Diversity provides prosperity and opportunity for all and allows for regulations. This is why we have monopoly rules in place. Whether they are enforced or not is another story.

This monopolizing of the seed marketplace has already caused major devastation in India where farmers used to plant their own seeds from the previous season's harvest. Monsanto came in and promised better yields with their seeds, and these poor farmers are now suffering. When a farmer buys the seeds from Monsanto, they also sign a contract saying

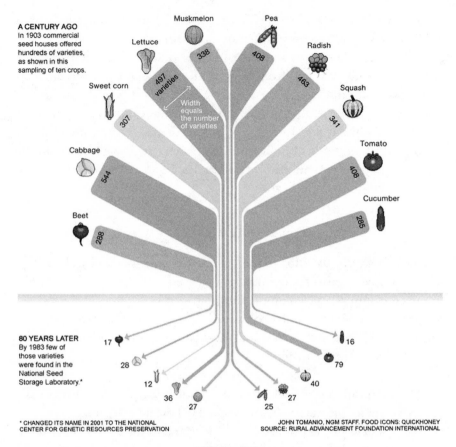

A CENTURY AGO
In 1903 commercial
seed houses offered
hundreds of varieties,
as shown in this
sampling of ten crops.

Muskmelon

Pea

Lettuce

Radish

338

409

Sweet corn

497
varieties

463

Squash

Width
equals
the number
of varieties

307

341

Cabbage

Tomato

544

408

Beet

Cucumber

288

285

80 YEARS LATER
By 1983 few of
those varieties
were found in the
National Seed
Storage Laboratory.*

17

16

28

79

12

40

36

27

27

25

* CHANGED ITS NAME IN 2001 TO THE NATIONAL
CENTER FOR GENETIC RESOURCES PRESERVATION

JOHN TOMANIO, NGM STAFF. FOOD ICONS: QUICKHONEY
SOURCE: RURAL ADVANCEMENT FOUNDATION INTERNATIONAL

Figure 5.3
Source: RURAL ADVANCEMENT FOUNDATION

they will pay royalties year after year with the harvest from the "second seeds." Many farmers experienced low yields because of weather and still had to pay the royalty fee. Sadly, many farmers went into debt and many committed suicide because they could not pay their debts.

How Do We Not Buy GMOs?

The expert opinion is about 70 percent of food on shelves (processed food) contain GMO ingredients and as of 2016, 92 to 94 percent of all corn, cotton, and soybean crops are GMO. Eating whole fruits, vegetables, and grains—not stuff that is mixed in and processed—is another way to avoid them because GMOs are produced and used in products as a filler. Also avoid eating meat because they are in animal feed.

The use of GMOs is something that should be looked at carefully and thoughtfully and go through many processes before hitting the market. This is not the case in the United States, and it is why you hear so many fights about it. Agriculture is a big business, but we are the consumers who buy it and fortunately many companies are listening. Use your voice. If you don't buy it, they won't make it. I would estimate we have all eaten GMOs no matter how careful we are, and we have no idea what the long-term effects are.

ORGANIC

Organic is a term used for food that has not been sprayed with certain pesticides. It pertains to food and if you see this on a label for meat, it means the animal was fed an organic diet.

I won't go into detail because you can find a full description of organic and the rules in Labels and Regulators, but here are a few things to consider with organic foods.

1. It does mean less pesticides were used, but it doesn't mean *no* pesticides were used. Organic produce has tested to have an average of 23 percent of pesticide residue, whereas conventional farming has 77 percent.[4]
2. Some farmers have much stricter practices and use no pesticides.
3. Organic does not mean the animals were grown humanely; it just means they were fed an organic diet.
4. Organic doesn't mean healthy when it comes to sugar. An organic candy bar isn't healthier than a nonorganic candy bar because the sugar is organic. It just means it was grown without pesticides. Just like organic tobacco still causes cancer like regular tobacco.
5. GMOs are prohibited in organic farming.
6. It is healthier for our environment; soil from organic farming is healthier than conventional farming using pesticides.

There are many articles on the nutrition of organic versus conventional food. I found the article, "Is Organic Better for Your Health? A Look at Milk, Meat, Eggs, Produce and Fish," from *The Washington Post*, to be extremely informative and factual.[5]

BIODYNAMIC FARMING

Biodynamic farming is the new trend in small farming that is rapidly catching on. Created by philosopher and scientist Rudolf Steiner in 1924, biodynamic farming is a holistic approach to farming, creating a stable ecological balance among land, plant life, animals, and human work and consciousness. The farm is seen as an organism with each part contributing to its wholeness and health. There are no pesticides used and biodynamic relies on crop rotation, compost, manure, minerals, and herbal preparations. Following nature's natural cycle and working with the land, not against it, are all part of biodynamic farming. To some, it is mystical, and to others it is simply listening and working in harmony with nature. For you the consumer it means no pesticides, and fortunately it is popping up more and more in grocery stores. Biodynamics is practiced in more than fifty countries worldwide with crops ranging from viticulture in France and cotton in Egypt to silkworm breeding in China. Germany accounts for nearly half of the world's biodynamic agriculture, and Demeter International[6] is the primary certification agency for farms and gardens using the methods. I get biodynamic tomato sauce from Italy at my local Whole Foods.[7]

SUMMARY

The issue of how to farm isn't cut and dry. Our world population requires we find ways to mass-produce foods. Not everything is scalable if we continue to eat the way we do.

The healthiest ways to eat include:

1. Minimal or no pesticides: The reduction of pesticides is healthier for you, the soil, and the farmers and workers who grow it.
2. Local and seasonal: Most of the "fresh" fruits and vegetables are trucked or flown in and could be a week from picking before they make it to your grocery store. It is healthiest to eat a vegetable within two days or less of picking. Although I certainly buy raspberries from Mexico during December in New York City, eating what's in season is less expensive for you and also helps support local farmers.
3. Dirt: Your food should have a little dirt on it. Our produce is picked and scrubbed and shined before reaching the stores. The dirt in soil

contains important microbes your body needs to have a healthy digestive system.

4. Heirloom: Nonhybrid seeds are bumpier, more colorful, less "perfect," and more nutritious than hybrids, which have been crop after crop to be redder, plumper, more resistant to time and travel conditions, and in turn, are less tasty.

5. Diversity: The grocery stores may have variety of fruits and vegetables but not necessarily unique plants that a local farmer will grow. My local farmer has wasong, burdock root, wild chamomile, and many other seasonal plants that provide the nutritional and health benefits we lost long after we industrialized everything.

I shop from local farmers whenever I can. I try my best to buy produce that is not just organic but is also local and hasn't been sprayed at all and is not GMO. I also buy the "ugly" stuff, which is usually more flavorful. Living on the East Coast is tough, and I do not eat turnips and potatoes all winter long, but I do eat more of them during the winter months. When I shop at my local grocery store, I always look for the origin, which is something I didn't do a few years ago. Travel time and distance is really important in getting the freshest foods. You want your food to be as close to living as possible for the most nutrition. Many colder climate farmers are using greenhouses to grow during the off season. This has many benefits; travel time being one of them.

A whole book could be written on whether organic, biodynamic, or conventional farming is best, and in fact, there are many out there. If you wish to delve in further, a few suggestions follow. I recommend reading and coming to your own conclusions. It may not be the most exciting read, but your food supply deserves thoughtful time and consideration. It is a complex issue, one that needs to be thought through, and it is definitely going to be an important topic as our population continues to grow, along with our health issues.

- *We the Eaters* by Ellen Gustafson
- *The Third Plate* by Dan Barber
- *Farmacology* by Daphne Miller
- *Bringing It to the Table* by Wendell Berry

CHAPTER 6

PESTICIDES AND BEES
What Is Happening to the Bees and Why Does It Matter?

OUR BEES are dying at an alarming rate. Former president Barack Obama put seven different species of bees native to Hawaii on the endangered species list in 2016. In 2017, the bumblebee was added to this list for the entire continental United States. The bumblebee was once abundant in twenty-eight states and is now found in limited amounts in only thirteen states. Since the late 1990s, the species has plummeted 87 percent. In 2016, 44 percent of the honeybee population died off.[1]

Why Is This a Concern?

Bees are key to our food preservation. Without bees to pollinate, we would lose many fruits and vegetables we take for granted, with 87 percent of crops benefiting from insect pollination according to an article from the United Nations' Food and Agriculture Organization.[2]

A chart of the species of bees and the foods they pollinate is available at Wikipedia.[3] Imagine losing strawberries, oranges, and lemons. Losing even one of these would be devastating, not to mention the loss of income for farmers.

So what exactly is killing the bees? There are many factors scientists and researchers are looking at. So far there are three that have garnered the most concern.

First, a class of pesticides called *neonicotinoids* have been shown to be a definite cause. Fortunately in 2017, before the Trump administration began dismantling the EPA, the Obama administration passed regulations about these neonicotinoids, regulating them.[4] The EU has restricted the use of these pesticides since 2013, a year after the study, "Existing Scientific Evidence of the Effects of Neonicotinoid Pesticides on Bees," came out showing how neonicotinoids were part of the bee populations' demise.[5] As of writing this chapter, the EU had completed an analysis on the current bee population in Europe, but it was not yet available for public review. Hopefully, we will see an increase from their efforts.

The next cause is weather. Bees may be synonymous with warmer weather, but they can't take significant heat. As the weather patterns become more erratic, the bees have not adapted with their migration, causing a loss in the species.

Finally, a tiny parasite called *Nosema ceranae* is the third cause attributed to the death of bees.

What scientists know is that a combination if all three of these has attributed to the demise of our bees. Unfortunately, no one cause can be pointed to as the exact reason. This real problem needs continuous observation and assessment by farmers, chemical suppliers, and scientists. It does no good to ignore the issue; the stakes are far too high. Although pesticides may provide an immediate relief for a farmer, there are no long-term benefits if the pesticides kill the very pollinators that bring the plant to life.

CHAPTER 7

SEVEN ITEMS TO KEEP AND SEVEN TO THROW OUT OR AVOID

IN MY JOURNEY of recovering from breast cancer, I took a long, hard look at my own food choices. I did not consider myself a bad eater, but of course I had room for improvement. I researched, read, and attended lectures on new foods that promise to bring us health and wellness. I widened my palette and started trying many different plants, spices, and elixirs. A summary of what I found and what resonated with me follows. Eating five pints of blueberries a day will not ensure you stay cancer free; nothing will. However, I think in our ever-increasing chemical-laden world, we need to take as many measures as we can to reverse the effects of the toxins we inhale every day. The foods that follow all have studies of their benefits and detriments.

SEVEN FOODS I EAT OR USE DAILY

1. Seaweed. I am a vegetarian who eats fish once or twice a week, so I do get a lot of my protein from the sea. This also means I am eating a lot of heavy metals found in our fish. Seaweed is a great source to detox from the metals because it acts like a sponge and soaks it up. This also means the seaweed soaks it up in the oceans, so I am careful of where I source mine from. It is relatively tasteless when mixed in

a morning fruit smoothie and is great in salads and soups. Seaweed has also shown to help gut flora and thyroid disorders and is high in lignans (antioxidants that support the immune system), which help to block the chemical estrogens that can predispose people to cancers. It provides a lot of minerals and has been shown to prevent high blood pressure in animals.

2. Vitamin D3. Hopefully you have a good doctor who has already put you on vitamin D supplements and monitors your levels in the winter time. Vitamin D3 is processed by everyone differently, so a blood test is the only way to make sure your levels are optimal. Proper levels of D3 reduces your chances of cancer and depression. Recent studies have shown that vitamin D deficiency is found in Alzheimer's disease and dementia, suggesting that having an optimal level would prevent both. I take a very high dose in liquid form because I do not absorb it easily. I also give it to both my husband and ten-year-old son.

3. Turmeric, cinnamon, and spices. Turmeric is a wonderful spice that has found its way back into our kitchen. A powerful anti-inflammatory, fresh turmeric is something I add to my morning smoothie daily. I also add it to my humus; I mix it in green juices, almond milk, smoothies, and so on. It has a light flavor and is not too overwhelming, making it easy to incorporate into your daily diet. The powerful phytonutrient found in turmeric—Curcumin—is activated by black pepper. To get the most from this spice, add some black pepper to enhance the anti-inflammatory effects. In addition to turmeric, I have widened my use of spices in every meal. I add cardamom and coriander to my morning smoothies. I use fennel for digestion and created a masala box containing nine spices I use weekly. Spices are powerful medicines and have long been used in natural healing for thousands of years. If you have blood sugar issues and eat a fruit or a sweet, add cinnamon, which is a powerful blood sugar regulator. I add cinnamon to my coffee every morning with a little honey.

4. Maitake and other mushrooms. If you want to know what to eat and what heals, have a conversation with your local farmer. This is how the magical maitake mushroom (also known as hen of the wood) came my way. One of my local farmers who has an impressive array of mushrooms introduced me to this healing fungus, and it is a weekly purchase

for me. It is high in protein, and studies have shown it to be a powerful glucose regulator. It is a power food for those concerned about type 2 diabetes or with blood sugar issues—something I personally have to watch. There have been many studies on this powerful mushroom, with several researchers corroborating that maitake causes apoptosis ("programmed suicide") of cancer cells and contains anti-angionenesis properties. See "Maitake: The Magnificent 'Dancing' Mushroom" at the *Huffington Post* website for detailed information.[1]

Note: All mushrooms are power sources and bring us many benefits. Mycelium extract (found in all mushrooms) is being heavily researched by pharmaceutical companies for its cancer-fighting properties, and many patients are already incorporating it in their treatment. Mycelium has been shown to not only clean up oil spills on land, but also regenerate and produce a new ecosystem when placed on top of the oil. It can be used as a natural pesticide, is a powerful antibiotic, and has been shown to treat flu viruses. I also take resihi mushroom extract, which has helped me tremendously with my blood sugar and tiredness.

5. Floradix. Anemia runs in my family and is a problem for many. After radiation treatment, my iron was so low, I had to do a colonoscopy to make sure I was not bleeding internally. Along with a family history of anemia and my plant-based diet, I was forced to look at this deficiency and find something to help quickly. In the past, I had tried iron pills, but suffered from constipation and had minimal increase in my iron levels. Then I discovered Floradix. Common in Europe and made in Germany, Floradix came recommended to me by my girlfriends. It is an herbal liquid that unlike traditional iron pills, once I started it my iron levels immediately increased. If you have anemia or are a vegetarian, try this. It does not cause any sort of constipation and comes in a vegetarian and vegan formula. It is also loaded with B_{12} and other vitamins. They also have a magnesium formula that is good as well.

6. Local raw honey. If you suffer from seasonal allergies, taking a teaspoon of honey daily can help you adjust to the local pollen. It is a sugar but an unprocessed one. Raw honey ensures all the nutrients remain intact and are not heated off.

7. Certified Humane eggs. One of the biggest fallacies going on is how egg-laying hens are treated on organic, pasture-raised chicken farms. Organic means they get organic feed. Pasture raised means they have some time outside on a pasture. What it does *not* mean is that they are treated humanely. This was a big revelation to me. You would be shocked to know the conditions of organic, pasture-raised chickens. Many have thousands of chickens in a barn—cage-free but crowded. They are so crowded that they saw off their beaks to prevent them hurting and pecking one another. Many do not even go out into the pasture, which is also small and crowded. The ammonia stench from their excrement is overwhelming to humans and chickens alike. In her book, *Farmacology: Total Health from the Ground Up*, Dr. Daphne Miller goes into great detail on the smell of "organic, pasture raised" egg farms she visited.

   Although not perfect, Certified Humane eggs mean they are treated humanely and is much closer to the vision of a happy chicken on the carton. Look for this seal at your market, or better yet, get your eggs from a trusted farmer who does not mass produce eggs but has a few hens and sells a dozen cartons a week along with produce.

   As a note, conveniences are not what they seem when it comes to food. Always get your fruits and veggies whole from the farmer or organic and frozen. The convenient cut-up lettuces and veggies in a bag are often "triple washed" with chemicals such as chlorine bleach or solvents like butoxypropanol, which was shown to be toxic to rats. If you buy it bagged, always rinse and clean it.

SEVEN FOODS I AVOID

1. Canola (Rapeseed), Corn, Palm, or Soy Oils. Like corn syrup, canola oil was created because of an abundance of the rapeseed plant in Canada in the 1970s. It has successfully been marketed as a "natural" oil, however natural doesn't mean you should consume it. Canola oil is used as a biofuel and a natural pesticide and the largest growers are Canada and China. Like corn and soy, most of it is genetically modified; 90 percent of Canada's canola oil is GMO. If frying something on high heat, I use sunflower oil, which

admittedly isn't great, but has no flavor like coconut oil, which is far better for high heat, but will leave its sweet taste behind. (Most vegetable oils are blends of canola, corn, and soybean oils). In general I avoid high-heat, fried cooking, and I stick with coconut or olive oil, which are pressed oils—not highly processed like most vegetable oils. Ghee, which is clarified butter, is also great for adding flavor, and you can use a lot less than regular stick butter and get an intensified butter taste.

What's the deal with palm oil? Palm oil is a great example of a good oil gone wrong. Palm oil is sourced from the seeds from palms, and like coal, it has good intentions, but we have oversourced and overused it with horrible consequences. The need for palm oil in processed foods is a major source of deforestation, pollution, habitat loss, and global warming (see http://www.wwf.org.au/what-we-do/food/palm-oil#gs.6fRszyg). Diversity and less industrialization of our food is a must to make sure this doesn't happen with other foods we tend to trend on and demand like coconut oil, chia seeds, and almonds, just to name a few.

2. White flour and nonorganic grains. I regularly bake with sprouted, whole wheat flour or spelt because white flour holds little nutritional value and also plays havoc with my blood sugar. Besides pie crusts, it has been easy to switch over. Buckwheat flour is now one of my favorites, and I prefer its earthy taste. For me, whole grain flours digest easier; I have less bloating; and I receive energy from it compared with lethargy and crashing blood sugar with white flours. When it comes to grains, organic and local is the best in my opinion, and if you can get heirloom grains, even better! Our wheat has been hybridized and changed over the years because of population growth and industrialization. Not only have our grains changed, but they also carry less nutritional value than what they once had. Much of it is also sprayed with pesticides, which not only stays on the plant when it is ground into flour but also stays in the soil. The USDA requires that a farmer must wait three years and use no pesticides on land he hopes to call organic. Just imagine how pesticides stay in the plant if it stays in the soil that long? Therefore, when I buy grains, I only buy organic ones. Fortunately, I am able to also buy stone-ground wheat that is grown locally—without pesticides.

Rice is heavily imported from China where they have lax regulations. If it is certified USDA organic, they do have to meet our guidelines, but who knows how monitored they are—particularly with the 2017 U.S. administration cuts on our regulators. I read all the labels and only buy organic rice that is grown in the United States. Soil health is extremely important with a crop such as rice, and I will pay the extra two dollars for local and organic. Gluten free is an option and many of the gluten-free versions are delicious. Be careful though because some are full of ingredients you normally would not consume large amounts of, like cornstarch.

3. Corn syrup, high fructose corn syrup, and white sugar. I do not buy anything with corn syrup. Corn syrup is a highly manufactured product that does nothing but harm to our body. It is added in so many things, including hamburgers, fish sticks, sodas, cereals, drinks, chips, cookies—even pasta sauce. Most pancake and waffle syrups are just corn syrup flavored with artificial maple. Its introduction into our food system is also aligned with the start of obesity in the United States, and in my opinion it should be banned. Fructose is found in fruit, but processed fructose or high fructose is a completely different product and is a highly concentrated form of a natural sugar. It is not satisfying and has been described as addictive, making the eater want to eat more and more. White sugar is something I try to avoid. I bake with coconut sugar or brown sugar (a lesser processed version) or pure maple syrup. Unsweetened applesauce is a wonderful way to add moisture and sweetness to baked goods.

4. Fake foods. Margarine, artificially flavored foods, fake cocoa chocolate, whipped cream made from vegetable solids (cool whip), low carb, and all synthetic sugars—aspartame (NutraSweet®), sucralose, acesulfame k, saccharin, and xylitol. I don't believe in a knight-in-shining-armor and I don't believe in substitutes for actual foods. It has been proven time and time again that they do not help you lose weight or fat or help your heart stay healthy. In fact, they often do the opposite. Food should not and does not need to be a chemical or altered. Your body is made to eat whole foods and does not know how to process chemicals.

5. Artificial Colorants. Most food colorings, except Blue 2 (which is indigo and approved for dying jeans as well as candy), are petroleum-derived products. Cosmetic colorants come from coal tar, but food grade

colorants are from crude oil. Although they can certainly add beauty to a frosting or bright orange colors to chips, they serve no purpose and are something our bodies were never meant to ingest. Many studies have linked ADHD and some to cancer. According to the report, "Diet and Nutrition: The Artificial Food Dye Blues," in *Environmental Health Perspectives*, McDonald's uses real strawberries to color their sundaes in the United Kingdom.[2] In the United States, they use Red 40 because they can. There are several natural colorants out there, such as saffron for yellow and beet juice for red. Thankfully these are becoming more and more available in grocery stores and bake shops.

6. Processed meats. I do not eat meat, but my husband and son still do. When buying sliced meats for them, I only buy those that have been cooked in the store and are in full animal form, not meats that have been pressed into a gelatinous cylinder. Those meats contain added salts, nitrates, gelatins, and preservatives such as MSG. It is also baked in plastic. A video on the process can be found at https://www.youtube.com/watch?v=RrmcO1QBEo8.

7. Milk. Although I do use milk in some cooking or baking, I do not offer it to my son for drinking and have dropped it from my coffee. We have fortunately evolved to a better dairy practice with no antibiotics being used in most milks, but we are still a long way off. Almond milk has twice as much calcium as milk and that along with coconut milk is what I use in my coffee or for my son's cereal. There are many who believe that we are not supposed to drink milk and that it is for the calves. I am not one of them. I think milk is okay in limited quantities. I think a little bit in a recipe is okay—personally I maybe have one-fourth cup a week. My issue is with how it is produced and how it affects us by drinking it. Dairy cows are kept in a lactating state. This means they have to be artificially inseminated and are kept pregnant. Their calves are taken away immediately and they are constantly being milked. Their lives are generally five years, but if they lived in nature without constantly being milked, they would live for twenty years. Although this may be a personal decision, I do believe the treatment of an animal and the quality of a milk we then drink is something to be concerned about. A recent study from Harvard also shows a higher risk of prostate and ovarian cancers from those who consume large amounts of milk.[3]

There is currently a surplus of milk because we are drinking less dairy. Dairy farmers dumped more than 43 million gallons of excess milk into fields, manure lagoons, animal grain, or elsewhere in the first eight months of 2016.[4] This is poor farm management at its best and such an incredible waste. The USDA stepped in and bought $20 million of cheddar cheese to help absorb the loss. And where does the cheese go? The "marketing group" for dairy farmers (paid for by dairy farmers) has lobbied and invested millions with McDonald's and Dominos and others to create more "dairy-heavy" menus. This means extra, extra cheese on your pizza and maybe some new cheese fries on the menu. Like corn syrup, your health and your family's health is never a consideration. It is *always* about profit.

I am aware of the difficulties of elimination—particularly with a family. Although my son and husband will argue this for themselves, I do not see this process as elimination, but that I am eating for my health and wellness. I battle daily with my son over candies and sweets and with my husband who holds a deep fondness for white flour. I don't always win, but if I am cooking (and I usually am) then they go along with it out of sheer laziness! I hope that over time they will come to adjust their taste buds and experience the deliciousness of hearty full grain bread, over a processed white baguette from the grocery store. I see my son making good choices and preferring the real "food," and I know it is sinking in. Personally, I would rather go hungry than eat a slice of store-bought white bread with processed meat. I know how awful my body will feel and the repercussions I will face with my blood sugar. That alone is enough for me to stay away, and I see my family realizing this, too.

There are wonderful recipe books out there, and cooking with health as your intention should not be difficult or challenging. It should be easy and fun and most of all delicious. Here are a few resources that have helped me in my own kitchen, particularly Detoxinista.com who makes it healthy and delicious.

- *The Gene Therapy Plan* by Dr. Mitch Gaynor, M.D.
- Detoxinista.com, which has wonderful, healthy recipes
- *Healing Spices* by Bharat B. Aggarwal

CHAPTER 8

MEAT AND FISH DEFINED

THERE ARE many layers to meat and fish consumption; it is a bit overwhelming so I have compiled a summary of the key points to get the conversation started. I urge you to visit the resources, and if you are lucky to have one, speak to your local farmer to make the choices best for you and your family.

MEAT

First let's look at commonly bought meat: beef, lamb, pork, chicken, and turkey.

Impact on the Environment

When considering your meat, sustainability is equally as important as the origin. Sadly, there isn't much sustainability in factory farming and beef is the worst. A third—33.33 percent—of our world's land (that is suitable for growing food) is currently being used for cattle production. It takes more than 5,000 pounds of feed and in excess of 4,000 gallons of water to take one—just one—beef cattle to its slaughtering age of twenty-one months. In comparison, a human being drinks one gallon of water a day; so for twenty-four months that would be 730 gallons versus the 4,000 for the one cow. Arguably we use a lot more to cook, bathe, and maintain hygiene with, but when it comes to drinking, that one cattle is outdoing us in water consumption by 75 percent. Animals raised for meat eat 60 percent of all grain produced in our world and there are still 925,000,000 humans going hungry and 884,000,000 who lack clean water. This is why you read or hear environmentalists asking us to reduce our red meat consumption; it simply takes too much of our resources.

Animal waste is another huge contributor to the detriment of our water—in this case, the pollution and contamination of it. Nitrogen and phosphorus are needed to keep soil healthy and manure does provide this; it is a natural fertilizer. But the amount of manure produced far exceeds our needs. One cow produces 65 pounds of manure a day and 3.5 gallons of urine.

In contrast, one thousand humans produce as much total waste solids as:

- 20 dairy cows or
- 60 beef feeder cattle or
- 280 feeder pigs or
- 6,200 laying hens or
- 11,000 broiler chickens[1]

It is an overwhelming amount, and all of this "waste" ends up somewhere. Currently farmers pool it in man-made "lagoons," which is a giant pool filled with poop. They frequently leak, and there are numerous cases of the "run off" contaminating local drinking water. In 2011 a runoff from a hog farm in Illinois killed 110,000 fish. This happens all the time. Agriculture runoff is 80 percent of the pollution of our water, with farm manure a significant contributor to the 80 percent.[2] The dumping of manure, pesticides, and fertilizer is killing our aquatic system, making beaches unswimmable and fish uneatable. It's as simple as someone plowing land and a rainstorm comes and the runoff goes into the water. Algal blooms are now a regular occurrence and are showing up all over our country. They are the result of excess nitrogen and phosphorus and come from agriculture runoff.[3]

This is not just beef, but pork, chicken, turkey, and lamb also contribute to this. One visit to a factory farm, even a large organic one, will be enough to put you off meat forever. Animals are often knee deep in their own feces, and you would find it hard to breathe inside a poultry house where the stench of thousands of thousands of birds produces an ammonia smell that is not only intolerable to you but also to the birds. Chickens actually have a sense of smell that is equivalent to ours.

Everyone has joked about cow farts killing our ozone layer, but sadly that joke is a real problem. The emissions of all livestock, not just cows, account for 35 percent of methane gasses released, and methane makes up 10 percent of the gasses eating our ozone layer. It is not as significant as the 82 percent of the complete pie from oil, natural gas, and coal, but it is definitely making an impact. None of this is made better by organic, grass-fed meat. They still belch, pass gas, make manure, and eat and drink the same as the nonorganic-fed animals do.

Deforestation

Animal agriculture is the number-one reason we are losing our forests. They are being cut down at a rate of forty-eight football fields a minute. And it is not for Ikea furniture. The deforestation is to meet the need and desire for meat.

Forests bring us immeasurable health via climate (the cutting of rainforests is a contributor to drought and less rain) and medicines for malaria, Hodgkin's disease, pediatric leukemia, cortisone, and antibiotics—with many yet undiscovered and still in trials. To destroy them to raise cattle and food for cattle—whose health benefits to us are questionable—is something we should all take a long moment to ponder.

Antibiotics

Antibiotics in animals have been commonplace for years. They are used for the many illnesses animals get because of the crowded and unhealthy conditions they are raised in, and a side effect is that it also makes them bigger. A chicken today is four times larger than a chicken in the 1950s and a chicken breast today weighs more than a whole chicken did in 1950. It is also why we may weigh more too. Antibiotics injected into animals stay in their flesh and then go into your flesh when you eat them or drink their milk or eat their by-products such as eggs and cheese. This small amount builds up over time and is one of the concerns or causes of human antibiotic resistance we face today.[4]

Animals are also becoming resistant to the antibiotics, which are not working on many diseases, and humans are now getting these diseases when they eat the sick animals' flesh. This is why well-cooked meat is extremely important. Fortunately, we do have antibiotic-free meat available to us if we can afford it, but there are no guarantees what we are getting when we go out to eat.

The EU and Canada have recognized this health concern, and many countries have banned subtherapeutic use of antibiotics. Unfortunately, the United States continues this practice—with the meat industry leading the way stating there is not enough evidence to ban them, although experts in the EU, Canada, and WHO disagree.

Many (including myself) opt for organic and grass-fed meats to feed our families, feeling it is the healthiest and more humane option. At high prices, one would hope they are getting the best they can; however, my idea of best was greatly redefined after I really investigated what grass-fed, organic meat is.

Although organic (not grass-fed) meats are free of pesticides and hormones, grass-fed animals can be eating grass covered in pesticide. I would hope that they aren't, but it is not a given if the meat is not organic, too. It is also important to eat meat that was not pumped with hormones or antibiotics for your health. So even with grass-fed meat, you want to make sure that the grass was pesticide free and that they are antibiotic free.

As far as grass versus grain-fed meats, grass is better for the cows because it is what they were meant to eat and digest. Grain is fed to them because it is cheap, plentiful, and makes them fat quickly as they cannot digest it (hence the weight gain). It is often painful for the animal as anyone who has had severe gas pain can attest to. Nutritionally grass-fed beef is leaner, with higher doses of omega-3 than grain fed (about 50 percent more), but it is still far behind fish—a rib eye has 37 milligrams of omega and a piece of tilapia has 134 milligrams.

For poultry, you want to get the antibiotic- and hormone-free meat. This is covered in the organic label, but some nonorganic brands will make this claim as well. Like beef, there may be slightly more omega-3 in organic chicken but no other nutritional difference.

Pork is the same as beef and chicken. Organic is slightly higher in omega-3 as well. You want to be sure again to buy only antibiotic- and hormone-free meat because pork carries the highest percentage of bacterial contamination of all three. Mass-produced pork is also one of the filthiest of industries and 25 percent of the workers suffer from respiratory issues.[5]

So, is meat good or bad for you? Studies show that a more veggie-based diet is healthier and that meat should be a condiment or limited to a serving of one-eighth to one-fourth cup.

Many people believe that a largely meat diet is healthy and the way of our cavemen ancestors. Opponents to that will say our cavemen ancestors weren't great hunters and had to live primarily on plants and seeds, and meat was a celebration and a rare occurrence—certainly not daily or even weekly.

What we do know is that a primarily plant-based diet can reduce the risk and reverse type 2 diabetes and not eating red meat reduces your risk for colon cancer significantly. The rest of the studies get murky. Some doctors (with books selling their own diets) have found plant-based diets reduce or reverse some prostate cancers, and there is some evidence it reduces heart disease.[6]

How to Detox

It is quite clear that eating less meat is healthier for the environment and will soon be a requirement if we do not curtail it by choice. By reducing intake and limiting red meat to once a week, we could make a significant, positive impact for our environment and the preservation of our resources. It also may contribute to better health, and it certainly won't hurt it. If you desire meat with every meal, try reducing it to condiment size—that small reduction will also make a huge difference.

Always make sure the meat is organic and hormone and antibiotic free; this is indeed healthier. If you are eating grass fed for more omega-3, note that the extra cost may not be worth the minimal increase of this fatty acid. Grass is what cows are meant to eat, but it does not mean that the animals are treated better.

Buy your meat locally and from a small farm if possible. Ask the farmer about how the livestock is raised and if you can visit. Knowing how your meat is treated, raised, and slaughtered will serve you well as a meat eater.

I also want to cover animal welfare because I know many who spend their money on expensive meats truly believe the animal was treated more humanely. This is a fallacy we need to be clear on. Organic and grass fed does not mean humane. Organic and grass fed are all big businesses now, and although the cow may eat grass outside, it can still be crowded and sleeping in its own filth. This is the case with chickens and most fowl. Many organic, free-range hens live a hellish life. The standards are vague and grass-fed or organic does not mean a happy or healthy life. Organic, grass-fed milk cows are still slaughtered for meat after they become overmilked and too weak to produce—generally five years, which is the same as a regular dairy cow. Meat does not magically appear in a brown wrapper or plastic wrap, and the slaughter of an animal is not ever pleasant. They all are killed and just because it is organic and grass fed does not mean it was done humanely. Here are some of the treatments organic and grass-fed animals are also subjected to.[7]

- There are no rules to protect organic male chicks in egg-laying operations. They can be ground up, gassed, suffocated, thrown into garbage bags, or disposed of in other unsavory ways.
- Organic poultry raised for meat are allowed to be kept under continuous lighting and are allowed to be excessively fed.
- Some organic dairy cows are allowed to be kept in confined and small spaces, and others are allowed to be kept tied up.
- Organic pigs may have their tails chopped off and their ears notched.
- There are no rules in place protecting young organic livestock from being taken from their mother.
- There are no rules to protect organic poultry from having their beaks clipped.
- Debeaking, dehorning, and castration without painkillers is allowed in organic production.
- There are no rules against rough handling or yelling at organic livestock.

- Organic dairy cows and organic egg chickens will eventually be killed for meat in most cases.
- There are no rules surrounding how an organic animal can be killed, meaning a producer—organic or otherwise—may kill livestock pretty much anyway they like, including head beating, boiling alive, shooting, and more.

There are a few sites on the pros and cons of meat eating that I found well researched and valuable.[8, 9, 10]

FISH

My personal diet is plant based with fish. There is nothing I love more than a plate of sushi, and sadly, this too has its consequences. Eating fish in today's world involves mercury, sea lice, plastic fibers in the flesh, depletion of resources, and human slavery. Here's a look at the obstacles this industry is facing and some solutions you can take to your own plate.

Impact on the Environment

Eighty-five percent of the world's fisheries are at or above their capacity. An increase of more than 20 percent from 2000. This means there needs to be strict rules and regulations if we are to keep fish on our plates because of this overfishing. The rules and regulations we do have in place nationally and internationally are broken daily. People do not look to the next twenty years or even the next two. When money is your only concern, you do not think if your kids will be able to eat a can of tuna in ten years, you think about how you are going to feed them tomorrow. This translates to an excess of 20 to 50 percent of our fish being caught illegally. And we are catching more than we need—nearly 2½ times more. Governments try to control this, but with an open and vast sea, it is not easy. They also provide subsidies to fisherman who are not making enough money because our seas are overfished, and the price they get for their fish is not enough to make a living. So the government helps them out and they continue to fish and we continue to overfish, instead of addressing the fact that we don't have enough to sustain this industry. According to the World Wildlife Fund, species that are over-fished and on the list to avoid are nearly every form of tuna—Skip Jack, Albacore (canned tuna), Yellowfin (sushi and restaurant), Bluefin (sushi). Waters that are significantly overfished are the Artic, California Gulf, MesoAmerican Reef, Southern Chile, and the Galapagos.[11]

Overfishing also affects the seas natural ecosystem. When we pull too many large fish from the seas for us to eat, they are not feeding on the smaller fish. With too many smaller fish, the ecosystem becomes out of balance, and we have more algal blooms, which means no drinking water for us, no swimming, and the killing of the entire ecosystem where the bloom is. We are also pulling fish from the mouths of animals that need them like seabirds, penguins, seals, and more.

This is all as a result of greed and, perhaps, the blind-sightedness of people who do not want to see the change in an industry that they once thrived in. If we do not set real limits and make strong efforts to regulate and police this industry, we will soon be dealt with a no wild fish situation and only have farmed fish.

Farming and GMOs

Farmed fish is a solution, but it is far from perfect and also guilty of greed by trying to breed too many fish in crowded conditions that cause illness, which translates to not-so delicious fish on your plate. Farmed fish can also be GMO farmed in the same waters as the wild fish are, and they can and do escape, breeding with the wild ones, which eliminates the once-wild species as we have known it.

The farmed-fish industry is just as guilty as the industrialized meat industry of adding antibiotics and vaccines to the fish to kill or prevent disease and adding pesticides to the water to get rid of sea lice, which happens because of the close quarters. Inevitably what starts out as a good idea, gets pushed beyond its maximum, and like a fish tank with too many fish in it, you end up with major problems.

Fish are meant to swim and have space; the farmed fish are grouped together and the sea floor under them is filled with their excrement and food waste. There is so much excrement that not even nature can clean it up with her natural bottom feeders who can't survive because of the filth. Unfortunately, this experiment is taking place in our seas because the farmed fish share the same waters as our wild fish, but are netted off. Norway produces 80 percent of farmed fish today, and China, Vietnam, Japan, and India also are major producers of aquaculture. Given China and India's current state of pollution, this gives me additional pause for concern.[12, 13]

GMO Salmon

Genetically engineered salmon is now on our plates, and at the time of writing this chapter, the United States had no laws to inform the consumer. You may have eaten it whether you wanted to or not. Known as AquAdvantage salmon, it grows twice as fast—allowing more fish to the market faster and money to be made quicker.[14] GMO salmon was created by inserting a growth gene into a salmon egg, thereby decreasing its growth stage from fourteen to sixteen months instead of three years. This super salmon is twenty years in the making, and as far as I could see, there have been no studies done to determine the effects on human health. The fish will be produced in tanks, landlocked with no access to the ocean in Panama and Canada. Should one get into the ocean, it could take over the entire wild salmon population—leaving it permanently exposed to GMOs. Time will tell if this science is a good advancement or a detriment to our health and ecosystem.

Mercury

Mercury is found in fish because of pollution. Oil spills, air pollution, and sediment from the burning of oil, garbage, and manufacturing settles into our waters and our fish eat it. Mercury is not something that "washes away," and if a fish eats it, we eat it. Mercury bioaccumulates in fish; so the larger the fish, the more the mercury accumulates, making them the perfect host. Mercury also bioaccumulates in humans. Reducing your exposure and eating of this heavy metal is a real concern. You should have your levels checked every year to know if you are on the high side or not. Canned tuna is a big source of mercury in our food and here are others you should remove or eat less of in your diet: bluefin tuna, walleye, king mackerel, marlin, bluefish, shark, swordfish, wild sturgeon, opah, and bigeye tuna. Also of concern, but to a slightly lesser extent, are orange roughy, Chilean sea bass, blue crab, lingcod, Spanish mackerel, spotted seatrout, wahoo, grouper, snapper, halibut, tile fish, rock fish, sable fish, and blackfin, albacore, and yellowfin tunas.[15]

Omega-3

A positive benefit to eating fish is the omega-3 gained. Significant in salmon and mackerel and oily fishes, such as sardines and anchovies, omega-3 is thought to bring you brain health and a host of other benefits such as lower blood pressure, reduce unhealthy cholesterol, reduce the likelihood of heart attack or stroke, reduce the development of plaque in arteries, reduce depression, and increase cognitive health. Of interest to me was an experiment that journalist Paul Greenberg took to see what a year of eating just fish and vegetables did to increase his omega-3; surprisingly at the end of the year, his levels did not increase significantly. I highly recommend his documentary *The Fish on My Plate* on fish farming and ways we need to proceed to keep the fish on the menu.[16]

If omega-3 and sustainability and less mercury are concerns for you, eat more sardines and anchovies; both are packed with omega-3 out of any other fish and have the least amount of mercury. They are overfished, but primarily to feed salmon—sardines and anchovies are ground up and made into a meal fed to them.

Other Factors: Human Slavery and Plastics

The fish our pets eat also come with severe consequences. Most U.S. pet food has some form of ground fish in it that is caught primarily in seas of Thailand. Many of these workers on the boats are human slaves from Cambodia. They are lured by "brokers" with promises of high-paying jobs and soon find themselves in a living nightmare. Often shackled in chains, by their neck, they are at sea for as much as a year—never seeing land, working eighteen hours a day, losing fingers and limbs, and never receiving a day's pay. All in "debt," they are told they owe for getting the hellish "job." This is not rare and it is not uncommon. The Thai government says it does its best to police this, but the ships are "untrackable" because they are so far out to sea and rarely dock. Instead they attach to a larger ship—give them their haul—and stay out on the ocean so as to never be caught. When they do reach land, the men are chained so they do not escape.[17]

Performance fleece and active wear are items nearly every person has in their closet. It is inexpensive, keeps you warm, and is easy to care for. Sometimes they are even made from recycled plastic, which gives the wearer a sense they are doing good while working out. Unfortunately, the tiny plastic fibers these garments are made of are polluting our water in large ways. The microfibers are too small to be caught in our septic system and make their ways into our waters, where our fish are now eating them. One microfiber jacket releases two grams (the weight of a paperclip in fibers) of fibers into the water when washed in a front loader—every time it is washed. A top loader is worse, with seven grams of fibers being released—from one jacket.[18] A study at the University of California did a comparison on fish from California's coast and fish off the coast in Indonesia; a third of both fish had foreign objects in them, but California fish had plastics in their flesh— tiny microfibers—whereas the Indonesian fish did not. The reason? Washing machines are still a luxury there, as is microfiber.[19] The most affected fish are the smaller ones that are eaten whole or shellfish like oysters and clams because the larger fish have bigger bellies making it less likely to be eaten by us.

Along with our clothing, personal care items like shower gels and face scrubs contain small little microbeads, which are made from plastic. These microbeads are also being eaten by our fish because they are so small our septic system does not catch them, and they never biodegrade. The United States has banned them in rinse-off products as of January 2017; however, they are still allowed to be used in cleaning products.

Countries that have banned them, or are in the process, are the United States, the United Kingdom, The Netherlands, Ireland, and Canada. They are allowed everywhere else.[20]

How to Detox

This is a little tricky, is far from simple, and depends on what you want to avoid.

If you want to avoid mercury, eat smaller fish like anchovies and sardines.

If you want to avoid plastics, avoid anchovies, sardines, and all shell fish—and eat bigger fish like salmon.

If you want to support sustainable fish that clean the water (but you end up eating some of the plastic they ate), try mussels, clams, and oysters; they naturally help keep our waters clean.

If you want to avoid fish caught by human slaves, don't serve your pets food with ground fish in it.

And lastly, if you want to avoid GMOs, you can eat everything except salmon that is not designated as wild caught.

Alas as a fish eater, I have made a significant decrease in my tuna and other mercury-laden fish. My own levels were high, and I have them done every year now with my physical. This means less spicy tuna rolls and fresh seared tuna from my local fish monger.

I also eat local fish wherever I am (unless of course someplace that is known to be polluted or recently had a nuclear power plant leak). In New York, I am fortunate to have Blue Moon fishery, whose owner Alex values sustainability and protection of the seas (as most small-business fishermen do). His fish is fresh and local, and I enjoy every bite and am happy to support another small business owner. He has fished for years and knows what's good, what is dwindling in supply, and what to stay away from. After writing this chapter I will significantly reduce the amount of salmon I eat, which is hard because it is a personal favorite, making sure what I do eat is wild. I am also making an effort to eat smaller fish such as sardines and anchovies, but not too many because the idea of microfibers in my stomach is even less appealing than mercury.

Local and wild—as with meat—is what we all want and ironically what we all had before industrialization. As Farmer Wendell Berry says: "What I stand for is what I stand on."—the earth, the sea, the air. We must take care of it and demand the businesses who are profiting from our land do their part.

CHAPTER 9

WATER

WATER IS our life source. We need to understand that without it we will not survive. The lack of care we give it is astonishing, considering its importance to us and our survival. Most of us think it will always be there in our tap, flowing free on demand. However nearly nine hundred thousand people are still thirsty in this world, often walking miles to reach a dirty water source that you wouldn't put your foot in. When you consider that one in three people in our world do not have a toilet, it is clear that we have much more work to do in conserving and managing our waters.

Seventy percent of our global fresh water is used for agriculture. The majority of water is used to raise livestock for meat and corn. Our food system is not local but global. Your fruits and tomatoes—especially in the winter—come from places where it is warm, like Mexico. Many of the world's economies are food- and meat-driven, and without water to sustain it, wars and famine will start. If Mexico doesn't have water, it will affect all of us.

According to a 2015 NASA report, thirty-seven of the Earth's largest aquifers (an aquifer is a groundwater source) are being depleted at a rapid rate. With twenty-seven of these (in the United States, France, China, and India) surpassing their replenishment-versus-usage ratio.[1]

Limiting our use of the freshwater or increasing our efficiency of its usage are two things we can do to solve this problem. Many small countries like Israel have already made great strides to conserve their freshwater supply, with 86 percent of their freshwater being recycled.

Israel is the size of New Jersey, and for large countries, it is more difficult and expensive.

There is hope, and simple steps like efficient irrigation could resolve a great deal of our water worries and actually increase our crop yields.

According to an article in *National Geographic*:

- More-efficient irrigation practices, such as drip and microsprinklers, can reduce the volume of water applied to agricultural fields by 30 to 70 percent and can increase crop yields by 20 to 90 percent.
- Drip irrigation is used on less than 2 percent of irrigated land world-wide.
- Reducing U.S. irrigation demands by even 10 percent could free up enough freshwater to meet the new urban and industrial water demands anticipated for 2025.[2]

The ways are there; we as a global community must demand our governments do their job to keep our water healthy and flowing.

One of our biggest fallacies and dependencies is on bottled or canned water. We think we are drinking to our health and not damaging the environment; this couldn't be further from the truth. There are BPAs and other harmful chemicals in bottled plastic water, and even aluminum cans are lined with BPA liners or water-based "varnish," which is the same varnish I used on my floors when I sealed them. Glass is the better choice; however, it is still taking water from our natural pools, which we need.

Tap water is ultimately what we all should be able to use without care or concern but as we all know too well, clean tap water is nonexistent. Even if it comes from a pure source, it is treated with chemicals like chlorine for bacteria, fluoridated (for 69 percent of the United States), and then it comes to us. The "good sources" we do have that are not polluted with pesticides from farm runoff or illegal dumping are being drained by corporations such as Nestle, who take our purest water, bottle it and sell it to us.

This is admittedly a snapshot of a large problem, but hopefully it will have you taking action and becoming a defender of our greatest natural resource. Here is a look at bottled water (plastic, aluminum, and glass) and tap water and how they impact our health and environment.

TAP WATER AND WELL WATER

Our tap water comes from "natural" resources. This can be reservoirs (surface) and aquafers and wells (ground). It is pumped out and treated at our area water treatment plant, removed of fish and sediment, treated for any bacteria, and fluoridated. It is then pumped to us, where it comes out of our taps. After we use it to take showers, flush the toilet, wash our hands, this same water goes back to the treatment plant for filtration and cleaning again. It is sifted of garbage, phosphorus and nitrogen are removed (both cause algal blooms), and then treated with ultraviolet (UV) light, ozone, or chlorine. Chlorine is usually used as ozone and UV light are not always effective. It is then pumped back to you again to drink, cook, and bathe in.

Understanding this process, you can then see that there is no pure water. Period. Our natural water sources are all affected by pollution. To say you have the purest tap drinking water is really a naïve and untrue response. Every water is polluted with something; animal waste, for instance, would be prevalent in the purest of streams that run down a mountain valley. But with our industrialized world, that pure stream is really a mirage. The pollution from our industrialized world is every-where, including the air that carries toxic particles that fall into our rivers and streams.

For many reasons—survival being one of them—we tell ourselves the water we drink is pure and clean. The idea of giving a glass of chemicals to our child or grandchild is certainly something to make you pause. But indeed, that is what we are doing. All of our tap water has some amount of chemicals, heavy metals, and bacteria. There is list from the EPA showing "acceptable" guidelines for toxins in tap water.[3] If this list were followed, we would be doing much better than we are. Water is regulated and tested by the local treatment plants, but they fail to catch things all the time. There are numerous examples of this in the past three years in Flint, Michigan, with lead contamination and in Perrysburg, Ohio, with agriculture runoff poisoning the water and the treatment plant not noticing it. Residents there could not even use water to wash their dishes. My own family was affected by this and was using only bottled water. Many drank from it before it was found— including pets. My family said that they knew of five dogs within a few blocks of one another with the same rare form of cancer who drank the tap water.[4]

Lead contamination is primarily because of the pipes. In the case of Flint, lead became prominent when the city switched from Detroit water, whose treatment plant adds phosphates to control corrosion, to a cheaper water from the Flint River, which did not treat for corrosion. The water was also more acidic, thereby eating the rust on the lead pipes that then dumped itself into the water.[5] Lead pipes are not unique to just Flint and are in many cities across the United States. Water is not tested at the tap level frequently; how many times have you tested your water at the tap?[6] And with no plans for the pipes to be replaced, to be sure you do not have lead in your water, you would need to do regular testing yourself.

Well water is also susceptible to the same contaminants groundwater is. Agriculture runoff and toxins all make their way into the well water too. Even fluoride is naturally found in some well waters. Testing for wells need to be done privately, which can be as high as $2,000 and often not done regularly in poorer rural areas.

Another toxin in our tap water is prescription drugs. Many of us don't give any thought to what we flush down the toilet or drain. How do you safely dispose of old medicines? Down the toilet of course. Seems safer than the trash. We all have flushed old medicines down the drain or even dropped them accidentally, along with other stuff we did not know how to dispose of. I believe most of us who did this had no idea the harms it caused—simple lack of education like most pollution.

According to a Harvard study, 80 percent of the water samples drawn from 139 streams in thirty states, had drug contamination.[7] This included antibiotics, antidepressants, blood thinners, heart medications (ACE inhibitors, calcium-channel blockers, digoxin), hormones (estrogen, progesterone, testosterone), and pain killers. Caffeine and chemicals found in fragrances were also in there. If you would like to have your water tested, the EPA has this hotline EPA Safe Drinking Water Hotline (800-426-4791) for a list of contacts.

With so many concerns about lead, agriculture runoff, bacteria, fluoride, and drugs it is no wonder many turn to bottled water—but is that really better? In short, the answer is no because it is the *exact* same water coming out of your tap. Bottled water does not come from a fairy spring none of us have access to. In fact it often comes from your own water source.

Bottled, Canned, and Boxed Water

Bottled water is a billion-dollar industry, and it is one of the biggest and unhealthiest scams going, with 55 percent of bottled water in the United States coming from our own natural spring reservoirs and the other 45 percent coming straight from the tap.

This is not a joke, and it is not an exaggeration.

Companies are taking *our* natural sources of water and selling it back to us. The number-one offender of this crime is Nestle—the company you probably know for chocolate is also a billion-dollar company whose primary source of income is finding natural water sources and reselling that water back to the people who get it for free in their own taps. One of these brands—Poland Spring—is using Maine Spring water, but it is also the same water residents get for free in their tap. Nestle pays for it right? Unfortunately no. They specifically seek out land and old laws (like the one in Maine, which was set up to help farmers) that state water is free to all who live there. Nestle built a plant there, so now it is free to them too. Make no excuses for them; they are raping the land and people of their natural resources. Their community improvements and jobs are like a cigarette company paying for a smoker's cancer medication. Nestle has hundreds of "researchers" out there looking for land that has pure aquifers and no laws restricting the taking of the water. They also do this in California where they paid the San Bernardino National Park and Forest $624 a year to pump out millions of gallons of water for its Arrowhead bottled water.[8] That is thousands of tanks of water that Nestle gets fifty thousand in retail dollars. It is a sin. The CEO of Nestle, Peter Brabeck, has publicly said on film that the idea that water is a public right is an "extreme thought."[9]

Nestle is banking on our water getting more and more polluted, and their bottled water—which is from our purest—will be their ticket to ruling the world for as long as it lasts, I suppose. In the case of their Pure Life water, which is sold in impoverished countries like India, they will still take our water, purify it, and make us pay for it again. The poor people of India cannot even afford the bottled water, and Nestle won't allow the residents near their water plant to use the purified water tap. I honestly can't think of anything greedier than selling the public its own water.

Here is a complete list of Nestle's bottled waters as of May 2017.[10]

- Aberfoyle (Ontario, Canada)
- Acqua Panna
- Al Manhal (Middle East)
- Alaçam (Turkey)
- Aqua D'Or
- Aqua Mineral (Poland)
- Aqua Pod
- Aqua Spring (Greece)
- Aquarel (Spain)
- Arctic (Poland)
- Arrowhead (United States)
- Baraka (Egypt)
- Buxton (United Kingdom)
- Calistoga (United States)
- Carola (France)
- Charmoise (Belgium)
- Ciego Montero (Cuba)
- Contrex (France)
- Cristalp (Switzerland)
- Da Shan YunNan Spring (China)
- Dar Natury (Poland)
- Deep Spring (California)
- Deer Park (United States)
- Eco de los Andes (Argentina)
- Erikli (Turkey)
- Frische Brise (Germany)
- Fürst Bismarck (Germany)
- Gerber (Mexico)
- Ghadeer (Jordan)
- Glaciar (Argentina)
- Henniez (Switzerland)
- Hépar (France)
- Hidden Spring (Philippines)
- Ice Mountain (United States)
- Korpi (Greece)
- La Vie (Vietnam)
- Levissima (Italy)
- Los Portales (Cuba)
- Minéré (Thailand)
- Montclair (Canada)
- Nałęczowianka (Poland)
- Nestlé Selda (Portugal)
- Nestlé Vera (Italy)
- Neuselters (Germany)
- Ozarka (United States)
- Pejo (Italy)
- Perrier (France)
- Petrópolis (Brazil)
- Plancoët (France)
- Poland Spring (United States)
- Porvenir (Chile)
- Powwow
- Pure Life/Pureza Vital/

Vie Pure
- Quézac (France)
- Recoaro (Italy)
- Saint-Lambert (France)
- Sainte-Alix (France)
- San Bernardo (Italy)
- San Pellegrino (Italy)
- Santa Bárbara (Brazil)
- Santa Maria (Mexico)
- São Lourenço (Brazil)

- Sohat (Lebanon)
- Springs (Saudi Arabia)
- Theodora (Hungary)
- Valvert (Belgium)
- Viladrau (Spain)
- Vittel (France)
- Water Line (South Korea)
- Waterman (China)
- Zephyrhills (United States)

The other 45 percent of bottled water is tap water that companies fill in bottles and sell back to you. True story. Brands like Aquafina® and Dasani˚ (Pepsi), treat regular tap water and bottle it up to sell to you.[11]

Because this is all coming from our tap water and natural resources, the same contaminants are in there, too; you are just paying for them to be packaged in a plastic bottle. A study by the Environmental Working Group found that out of the ten bottled-water brands tested, thirty-seven chemicals were found, including coliform bacteria, caffeine, the pain reliever acetaminophen, fertilizer, solvents, plastic-making chemicals, and the radioactive element strontium. I tested a bottled water from a local drugstore, and it came up positive for pesticides. Bottled water is *not* necessarily safer.

Another issue is the plastic the water is sitting in. Most plastics, including water bottles, contain BPAs and phthalates that leach into our water. Phthalates and BPAs are endocrine disruptors that affect our health in so many ways: our weight, hormones, and sexual function, including conception. Our tap water is monitored for phthalates, and they are allowed in limited amounts. They should be removed in my opinion; however, bottled water isn't even monitored. According to the NRDC, "the bottled-water industry waged a successful campaign opposing the FDA proposal to set a legal limit for these chemicals." This means the water you are buying and that you think is healthier could actually be supplying you with unhealthy amounts of BPAs, phthalates, and even pesticides with each sip. Heat also boosts the amount of BPAs and phthalates released. If that bottled water bottle is sitting in the sun or stored in a warm warehouse (many are) or a hot car trunk, that is like food for phthalate and BPA productions. Most plastic bottled anything—water, soda, juice—is not free of BPA or phthalate, nor are the plastic cups and glasses you buy to use outdoors or by the pool. And many of the products claiming to be BPA free are not free of BPAs at all.

The government knows this; they even produce reports like this.[12] Every plastic has some chemical in it leaching in our water. A list of chemicals can be found in the article "The Truth about Plastic Water Bottles."[13]

1. Polyethylene terephthalate (PETE or PET). It is used for most water and soda bottles. The ingredients include resins made from methane, xylene, and ethylene combined with the chemical ethylene glycol and other chemicals. These have flame retardants and UV stabilizers added.
2. High-density polyethylene (HDPE). It is used for milk and water jugs and opaque food bottles. Resins made from ethylene and propylene resins and have flame retardants added. When burned these release formaldehyde and dioxin if chlorine was used during manufacturing.
3. Polyvinyl chloride (PVC or V). It is used in some cling wrap, soft beverage bottles, plastic containers, plumbing pipes, children's toys, vinyl windows, shower curtains, shades and blinds, and many other items. It creates toxic by-products when burned such as PCBs and dioxins. It is made from petroleum resins and has flame retardants added.
4. Low-density polyethylene (LDPE). It is used in plastic grocery bags, plastic wrap, bubble wrap, dry cleaning bags, and flexible lids. Resins made from ethylene and propylene resins and have flame retardants added. When burned, these release formaldehyde and dioxin if chlorine was used during manufacturing.
5. Polypropylene (PP). It is used in yogurt cups, some baby bottles, screw-on caps, toys, and drinking straws. Resins made from ethylene and propylene resins and have flame retardants added. When burned, these release formaldehyde and dioxin if chlorine used during manufacturing.

6. Polystyrene (PS). It is used in egg cartons, foam meat rays, clear take-out containers, plastic cutlery, toys, cups, and CD containers. Resins made from ethylene and propylene resins and have flame retardants added. When burned, they release styrene and polyaromatic hydrocarbons.
7. Other (usually polycarbonate). These are used in five-gallon water bottles, some baby bottles, and lining of metal food cans. They create toxic by-products when burned such as PCBs and dioxins. They are made from petroleum resins and have flame retardants added.

Why is this allowed? Because we buy it. The bottled-water industry is a $12-billion industry annually, and we all support it every single time we purchase a plastic bottle of water.

What about Canned Water?

Canned water is not any better. I have always opted for canned water over plastic, but it makes no difference. Canned beverages—water, soda, and beer—are all lined with BPA varnish to keep the can from corroding.[14] Hopefully by the time this comes to print there will be BPA-free canned beverages like there are BPA-free canned vegetables. The technology is there; the issue is acidity and not all food or drinks are able to be canned without erosion of some kind.

What about Bottled Mineral Water?

Mineral water—like spring water—is pulled from the source. Its high content of minerals and natural effervescence legally makes it mineral water. Sadly, it too is pulled from natural sources, then purified, which involves stripping it of all of its natural minerals, and then recarbonating it. As you can see from the list, Nestle has successfully purchased many of Europe's top mineral water suppliers as well. If it is in plastic, it is also getting BPA and phthalate exposure.

What about Home Filtration Systems?

Home-water filtration systems would seem the best option. They can successfully remove many contaminates. The issue is that they strip the water of everything, including the minerals that are good for you. Many people get sick after they install a water-filtration system because the minerals they need, like magnesium and calcium, are no longer there. Newer systems readd the minerals but not all of them. pH level is also important and should be tested if you have a water-filtration system. You want your body to maintain alkalinity for overall health. Simple water charcoal filters remove most impurities with the exception of lead and heavy metals. Reverse osmosis takes a tremendous amount of energy, using four liters of water to make one clean liter of water, and it is not that effective at removing bacteria. Ion exchange removes valuable minerals like magnesium, and boiling water simply doesn't appear to do a better job than a charcoal filter. Only reverse osmosis and distillation remove fluoride, and the amount is entirely dependent on your system. See http://www.explainthatstuff.com/howwaterfilterswork.html for more on this topic.

What about Boxed Water?

The newest trend to hit the market is boxed water, which is a box like a milk carton filled with purified water. The liner—like milk cartons—is lined with LDPE. This is a plastic that has shown minimal concern and is BPA and phthalate free, but still a plastic. Boxed water is a great idea in theory; however, the methods to make these cartons require more resources than plastic. Boxed water uses forests grown to make paper, but paper-making requires large amounts of water and chemical bleaches. Like plastic, paper requires a lot of resources to recycle and most towns do not have the facilities to recycle the cartons, so they just end up in a landfill. Glass also requires energy to recycle, but it takes a lot less energy to sanitize it and reuse it. Note: The water in the boxed brand I researched was purified water from a municipal source, meaning it was tap water, purified and then resold. Reusing materials is the optimal choice.

WHAT IS ADDED IN OUR WATER?

The guidelines of what our tap water can have in it and their limits are set by the EPA, *but* how they do it are up to your local water treatment plants. It is important to read your water report and know your water treatment plant. Google them and see if there are any violations on their part. Many things are added to our water, but you will need to ask them to know what is in yours. One ingredient to look out for is chloramine. This is a combination of chlorine and ammonia. Water protector Erin Brockovich wrote about chloramine in 2012.[15] To check your water, use this link that conveniently lists it, https://www.dudegrows.com/watercheck/.

WHAT CAN WE DO?

First and foremost, we all need to personally take action on this. Big business will continue to take our water, and the local government will continue to put our health aside until we say no. Check your local water and know what is in yours. I think it is worth it for everyone to have their water tested for lead. Lead will rarely come from your municipal supply, but rather from the pipes and everyone's pipes are different. If your water is bad, you need to demand your local officials clean it up. Call your local newspaper and go to town hall meetings. Reach out to waterkeeper.org, who do a fantastic job, with limited resources, protecting our water.

Personally, I cook and drink out of my tap water, and I drink bottled Mountain Valley Spring water in glass. In my research, this is the only source I have found to be pure from the spring that is unadulterated and privately owned. The pH average is a 9 and the fluoride content is below 0.1. The EPA fluoride limit is 4.0 and in New York City, where I live, it is 2.2. If I were unable to use my tap water, I would use Mountain Spring exclusively, which is delivered in glass jugs. Many have reverse osmosis, but I am not 100 percent supportive of reverse osmosis because it uses a tremendous amount of energy and wastes three liters or more to make one good liter of water.

In a perfect world, we would have much stronger laws to protect our natural water supply, allowing for us all to drink from our taps without concern and removing the need for bottled water. Our towns and cities would have working public taps and fountains for us to fill up our metal or glass travel bottles, and those mega companies who sell our water would be charged a proper rate—not get it for free—with that money going to keep our pipes and water treatment plants up to date.

It is entirely possible and also entirely up to us to enforce it. I am afraid there is not a consciousness in the big business of water, and the change will have to come from the demands and actions of the public at large.

CHAPTER 10

COOKWARE, STORAGE, AND COMPOSTING

HOME COOKING is the healthiest option for us all. Even if we love butter, we generally use far less salt, oil, and sugar than a restaurant. How then can we ensure the food we take so much care to buy is not being tainted with metals and toxins when cooking?

This chapter looks at how we cook our food, store it, and dispose of it and the safest options we have.

COOKWARE

Aluminum

Aluminum is the best conductor of even heat and is cheap and plentiful, making it an obvious choice for cookware. It did, however, raise a red flag several years ago when the autopsy reports of people with Alzheimer's disease showed high levels of aluminum. Aluminum is found in our soil, and it naturally transfers to plants. Medicines such as antacids contain a high amount of aluminum—more than 100 milligrams—with the average adult consuming 7 to 9 milligrams daily from food. *Cook's Illustrated* (https://www.cooksillustrated.com/how_tos/6390-cooking-with -aluminum-pans-controversy) did an in-house test on aluminum pans, cooking an acidic tomato sauce in the pot for two hours, and then storing the sauce in the same pan over night. Only 0.0024 mgs of aluminum were found to leach into the pot. Aluminum is a real concern and is a neurotoxin; although it doesn't appear to leach hardly anything, I also don't think a small amount serves us any good either. I use stainless steel pans with an aluminum core, these conduct heat well, but the aluminum is not leached into the pan. Taste wise, aluminum can also leave a metallic taste behind, particularly with acidic foods like tomatoes and lemons.

Nonstick Pans

Nonstick pans are made with a coating that admittedly gives off toxic fumes at temperatures above 500 degrees F. If heated above 660 degrees, they release fumes strong enough to cause flulike symptoms in you and death in a pet bird, whose respiratory system is much more fragile.

Above 600 degrees sounds *really* hot right? Not really. A good steak sear is at 656 degrees.

Here is a temperature gauge from *Good Housekeeping*. If you use Teflon nonstick pans, you may want to use them just for eggs.

Sticking Point

How fast will a nonstick pan reach 500 degrees F, the point at which its coating can start to decompose? The Good Housekeeping Research Institute put three pieces of nonstick cookware to the test: a cheap, lightweight pan (weighing just 1 lb., 3 oz.), a midweight pan (2 lbs., 1 oz.), and a high-end, heavier pan (2 lbs., 9 oz.). We cooked five dishes at different temperatures on a burner that's typical in most homes. The results: Even we were surprised by how quickly some of the pans got way too hot. Check out the test details (Table 10.1).

Copper

Copper has become a trendy pan to cook with and is favored by chefs because of its ability to conduct heat quickly and evenly. Copper pans should be lined with tin or steel—silver on the inside and copper on the outside. An unlined pan can leach copper into the food, and although we need a little copper in our diet, too much can be toxic. Copper pans look

Table 10.1

SAFE	RISKY
Scrambled eggs 218° F Cooked on medium for 3 minutes in a lightweight pan	Empty pan, preheated 507° F Heated on high for 1 3/4 minutes in a lightweight pan
Chicken-and-pepper stir-fry 318° F Cooked on high for 5 1/4 minutes in a lightweight pan	Pan preheated with 2 Tbsp oil 514° F Heated on high for 2 1/2 minutes in a lightweight pan
Bacon 465° F Cooked on high for 5 1/2 minutes in a medium-weight pan	Hamburgers 577° F Cooked on high for 8 1/2 minutes in a heavyweight pan
	Steak 656° F Cooked on high for 10 minutes in a lightweight pan

SOURCE: http://www.goodhousekeeping.com/cooking-tools/cookware-reviews/a17426/nonstick-cookware-safety-facts/

beautiful but are also expensive and a pain to polish. If you have them, use table salt and vinegar to scrub the outside to a coppery shine to avoid toxic chemicals on your pan.

Stainless Steel

Stainless steel is predominant in most kitchens and is also in my own. They often have copper or aluminum bottoms to help with even heat conduction. A study from 2013 found there was significant leaching of nickel and chromium from cooking with stainless steel.[1] And an excellent article from a researcher and consumer advocate Debra Lynn Dadd also confirmed the study that nickel and chromium are leaching when we cook.[2]

It does appear that after multiple uses, the leaching of nickel and chromium is reduced but still detectable.

Cast Iron and Enameled Cast Iron

Cast iron is great for me because I have an iron deficiency that I have to tend to daily. Cast iron definitely leaches iron onto the food, and if you are concerned about too much iron, these are not the pans for you. I have several and my only complaint is their weight. With more acidic foods like lemon and tomato sauce, the iron can alter the taste, although I have never had this issue personally. Besides iron leaching, there are no health concerns.

Cast iron pans can stick, but enameled cast iron stops that. If you don't mind the heaviness, but like how a cast iron pot cooks, try these. The enamel can chip, although you can still use the pan—unlike enamel over aluminum. Make sure to buy your enamelware from a company that has tested them in accordance with California's Prop 65 law. This will ensure that the enamel does not contain cadmium or lead, which are common in enamels overseas and are not monitored. The limit for cadmium in enamelware is 0.5 ppm, and for lead 90 ppm per the FDA. Le Creuset and Lodge brands both manufacture enamelware and state that their products meet FDA and Prop 65 requirements. However, blogger Natural Baby Mama had her house tested for lead and her Le Creuset pans had lead and cadmium—above the limits. The issue seems to be the color red because her blue enamelware all tested fine.[3] When buying enamelware, I will no longer purchase the red color. I will add that under the Prop 65 law, the onus is on the manufacturer. California has the law but does not test the products unless a red flag is raised by consumers.

Ceramic Ware and Stoneware

These products are used in the oven or microwave but cannot be used on the stovetop. The same concern with lead and cadmium applies here. These two heavy metals are found frequently in glazes used with stoneware. You can do a Google search and will find there are many countries who regularly ship in ceramic ware that violate the limits allowed. I would tread lightly when purchasing ceramic ware and would *not* use any ceramics purchased abroad for food. I have many beautiful bowls from Morocco that I use for decorative purposes, and as much as I wanted to bring home a tagine, I googled and read how some people had to throw theirs out after using because of the high lead content. This is not just Morocco, but Mexico, China, Japan, and even the United States for that matter.

Silicone

Silicone is a nontoxic product that is becoming quite popular in baking. It feels like a mix between rubber and plastic and is lightweight and flexible. It is frequently found in the form of muffin trays, baking mats, and oven mitts. It does not biodegrade; so if you use it, use it well. It can be recycled, but you need a recycling plant that works with silicone and that is unusual given the low demand. There have been no studies reporting the leaching of fumes or chemicals from these products and they appear safe, but they are also relatively new to the market. Some users have reported smells and smokes from use. I personally do not use them because I don't like how they handle and feel too flimsy for me.

Glass

Glass is an excellent option for baking; however, some cooks complain that it does not conduct heat as well as stone or metal for something like a pie. I remember my grandmother purchasing a new electric stove to use the "new" glass pots that came out. I cook with gas, which glass pots are not recommended for; however, this is a viable option for electric stovetops.

Slow Cookers

The pot of a slow cooker is ceramic/stone, and before purchasing, you should check the brand for lead safety or do a *Consumer Reports* search. Given you will be slowly cooking your food in the pot for six or more hours, I think it is worth the extra groundwork.

Lead Testing

If you are unsure like I was about lead in some of your cookware. I recommend testing them. A simple and reliable swab can be purchased online and you will have peace of mind. The down side is many of these tests have a false-positive from what I could find and are not as reliable as one would hope.

Storage

You should always store your food in glass. If glass is not an option, then stainless steel (don't microwave this obviously). The last option should be BPA-free plastic. According to a recent study cited in *Mother Jones*, even BPA-free plastics leached estrogen disruptors.[4]

COMPOSTING: IS IT WORTH THE EFFORT AND DOES IT HELP?

Composting is definitely worth the trouble because it reduces our waste in landfills. In most cases, waste sits in garbage bags, held in by plastic, taking decades to decompose. When you compost, you are reducing the methane gas emissions from our landfills, which in the United States are more than 20 percent of all methane gases emitted. One fourth of our food waste are yard and vegetable scraps, which is a considerable amount, therefore, we should all try to reduce by composting. In a city it is not easy, but fortunately more and more major cities have composting locations. A great article to help can be found in *Grist*[5] and also check with your local farmers market.

PART III

DETOX YOUR CLEANERS

I T IS EXCITING to me to see the progress we have made in using more natural cleaning products in our homes. From my own handmade creations off my stove to twenty years later, good options are readily available at nearly every grocery store. However, along with this great progress, there are great changes that still need to be made.

First our need to bleach, sanitize, and kill all bacteria is actually killing us and our immune systems. We are literally harming ourselves with daily use of hand sanitizers and products that are stripping away the immune system nature gave us. The second concern is regulation of ingredients. The cleaning industry, along with the beauty/makeup industry, is still unregulated for the most part. Ingredient disclosure is not required, and unless it is a pesticide or makes a claim "will kill 99 percent of germs," there is no testing required. Safety is based on the knowledge we have on individual ingredient testing. However, some unscrupulous person could put a bottle of formaldehyde mixed with water on a shelf and sell it as soon as the label was hot off the press.

The FDA is also extremely slow to investigate products. Take Tide for instance. Several years ago, a nonprofit group As You Sow were successful in getting Tide to reduce the percentages of 1,4-dioxane, a known carcinogen that is a product of ethoxylation, in its detergent. In real words, the soap is processed, and when it is processed, it produces 1,4-dioxane as a by-product. A natural comparison would be buttermilk which is a by-product of cream processed into butter. The FDA and EPA allow low levels of this carcinogen but rarely check to see if anyone is exceeding the levels. The state of California created their own law to fix this oversight called Proposition 65. Prop 65 requires manufacturers to disclose anything that exceeds the governmental threshold for carcinogens in a product. The Tide Free & Clear had levels of 89 ppm. By way of the Proposition 65 law, As You Sow, was able to get Proctor and Gamble to reduce its levels of dioxane to less than 25 ppm.

For those who believe this is rhetoric and that 89 ppm compared with 25 ppm is insignificant, animal studies suggest that daily exposure to 1,4-dioxane at concentrations above 50 ppm for two years caused liver and kidney damage. So consumers who thought they were using the purest form of Tide—with no fragrance, most likely on their children's clothing or those who are allergic to scent or have asthma—were actually wearing clothes on their skin that had residue of carcinogens. Perhaps it is harmless, but with one in two men and one in three women getting cancer in their lifetime, I would like to have full disclosure of what I am exposing myself and my family to—even if it is just detergent.

Fortunately, most companies have morals, and if you don't you have morals, you have a fear of a lawsuit or brand reputation loss. However, this does not mean that the government-allowed level is okay and because the FDA or EPA doesn't check, who is going to know? This also happens in the "natural" section where I see brands purposely omitting ingredients to seem better.

If no one is checking, the safest guarantee of a clean product is to make it yourself from pantry ingredients. This isn't always convenient, and honestly, sometimes more than natural is needed.

In this section, the chapters will take a look at all the options, explain to you the ingredients, and help you to make the best choice for you and your personal level of exposure to chemicals.

I do not preach someone should or should not use something, but I do believe that there should be full disclosure so you know exactly what you are using and exposing yourself to daily.

Let's get started.

CHAPTER 11

LAUNDRY

We all love fresh clean laundry. Perhaps nothing says love and caring for your home more than clean-smelling sheets or a sweatshirt fresh out of the dryer. Laundry is something most of us do daily, and the average American generates 500 pounds of laundry every year. This translates to 45 billion loads of laundry. 1,100 loads are started every second, and all those loads use 560 billion gallons of water, equal to the amount of water that flows over Niagara Falls every eleven days.[1]

And that is just the United States.

This is overwhelming, so let's tackle this in simple steps and suggestions.

First, we will look at how doing "the wash" affects the planet we live on.

LAUNDRY DETERGENT

Impact on the Environment

Ninety percent of the total energy used by a typical washing machine is to heat the water; only 10 percent is used to power the motor.[2]

Forty-nine percent of laundry loads run with warm water in the United States, 37 percent are run with cold water, and 14 percent are run with hot water.[3]

Thirty-four million tons of carbon dioxide emissions would be saved if every household in the United States used only cold water for washing clothes.[4]

Other benefits of cold water include less fading of dark-colored clothes, less shrinkage of natural fiber clothing, clothes last longer, and it works better on protein stains like blood. If you have workout clothing with odors, the addition of borax (a natural mineral powder) or a half-cup of white vinegar will take it out. Honestly, I rarely use hot/warm water.

By using cold water you reduce 350 pounds of carbon dioxide a year from being emitted. This reduces your personal carbon footprint by 0.05 percent a year. Perhaps this doesn't seem significant, but like crowdfunding, if we all contribute, we will make a big difference.

Half a ton of carbon dioxide emissions could be saved by line drying your clothing. If you can, you should. See my suggestions for fabric softening because line drying can make clothes stiffer.

Most of us now have high-efficiency (HE) machines; however, by using a front loader instead of a top loader, you can save an additional 7,000 gallons amount of water per year.[5]

car·bon foot·print *noun*

noun: carbon footprint; plural noun: carbon footprints

1. The amount of carbon dioxide and other carbon compounds emitted as a result of the consumption of fossil fuels by a particular person, group, etc.

cli·mate change *noun*

noun: climate change; plural noun: climate changes

1. A change in global or regional climate patterns, in particular a change apparent from the mid- to late twentieth century onward and attributed largely to the increased levels of atmospheric carbon dioxide produced by the use of fossil fuels. 2. A gradual increase

in the overall temperature of the Earth's atmosphere generally attributed to the greenhouse effect caused by increased levels of carbon dioxide, chlorofluorocarbons, and other pollutants.

Impact on Aquatic Life

Detergent runoff from "regular" brands like Tide are something to be concerned about. According to Lenntech.com, a company used by Shell, Chevron, and Coca Cola to clean up messes, detergents can have poisonous effects in all types of aquatic life if they are present in sufficient quantities, and this includes the biodegradable detergents. All detergents destroy the external mucus layers that protect the fish from bacteria and parasites, plus they can cause severe damage to the gills. Most fish will die when detergent concentrations approach 15 ppm. Detergent concentrations as low as 5 ppm will kill fish eggs. Surfactant detergents are implicated in decreasing the breeding ability of aquatic organisms.[6]

Always make sure to do full loads and not half-loads or less. Although our machines can use less water because they sense the size and weight of the load, the detergent is the problem here. Less wash, means less detergent in our water system.

To avoid 1,4 dioxane contamination, use detergents that are SLES or sulfate free. Our tap water has levels of dioxanes in it—most likely from all the sulfate soap we use—not just in detergent, but in shampoo, toothpaste, and shower gel.

Impact on Your Health

If you think all laundry detergents are created equally, try washing your clothes in my Good Home detergent and then do a load in Tide®.

I have not used Tide or another detergent in years, but recently I had to do a performance comparison and I was astounded by what I found.

The fragrance of the Tide alone made me want to throw the shirt out. Keep in mind, I am a fragrance person. I have won awards for the scents I created, but not all fragrances are created equal. I like to say you can smell quality. This scent is clearly made to stay on clothes and nothing else. It was so strong I could hardly stand it, and I knew if I actually wore the shirt laundered in it I would get a headache.

Next, the coating on the shirt from the "soap" was visible. It left an oily sheen that when placed next to the exact same shirt washed in my sulfate-free detergent looked like a polyester fabric when in fact it is 93 percent cotton.

There is no reason in this day and age we need to use detergents packed with chemicals. It is not healthy for us or our clothes; it does not make them "cleaner"; and it pollutes our waterways.

If you are still not convinced, here are the ingredients of Tide taken directly from their website; my notes are listed after the ingredients.

Tide HE ALL SCENTS
INGREDIENTS BY PROMINENCE
- water
- alcohol ethoxy sulfate: This is flammable, can cause skin and eye irritation, and is known to cause cancer in animals; see MSDS at http://www.colonialchem.com/fullpanel/uploads/files/colonial-ales-60-sds.pdf.
- linear alkylbenzene sulfonate: There is an environmental concern because it is toxic to aquatic life (and is the third ingredient in Tide).
- alcohol ethoxylate
- citric acid
- ethanolamine: There is a human concern because it causes severe skin burns, eye damage, and is found in oven cleaners and drain openers (and is the sixth ingredient in Tide).
- sodium fatty acids
- diethylene glycol
- propylene glycol
- sodium hydroxide
- borax
- polyethyleneimine ethoxylate: This material is extremely destructive to tissue of the mucous membranes and upper respiratory

tract, eyes, and skin. It has been known to cause spasms, inflammation and edema of the larynx and of the bronchi, pneumonitis, pulmonary edema, burning sensation, cough, wheezing, laryngitis, shortness of breath, headache, and nausea.

- ethanol
- protease
- sodium cumene sulfonate
- diquaternium ethoxysulfate: There is an environmental concern because it is found in the water system and is not biodegrading.
- Laureth-9
- fragrance
- amylase
- diethylenetriamine pentaacetate (sodium salt)
- disodium diaminostilbene disulfonate: There is an environmental concern because it is found in the water system and is not biodegrading.
- sodium formate: There is an environmental concern because it is found in the water system and is not biodegrading.
- pectinase
- calcium formate
- mannanase
- Liquitint™ Blue
- dimethicone: There is an environmental concern because it is found in the water system and is not biodegrading.

How to Detox

Hopefully, I have you convinced that you need to no longer use detergents that do not list their ingredients. Here are my suggestions.

1. Throw out and do not use any detergent that does not list its ingredients on the bottle. There is a reason they are not listing the ingredients. You can Google them and see; all major brands I checked contain petrochemicals and ingredients that are harmful to aquatic life.

2. Do not use a detergent with sulfates. See dictionary for specific names. But label should say sulfate free. Sulfates are not good for aquatic life and can be contaminated with high levels of 1,4-dioxane. Sulfates also deteriorate your fabrics and make them fade quicker.
3. Look for ingredients using cocamidopropyl betaine, sodium coco sulfate, cocamidopropylamine oxide, lauryl glucoside, and laureth-7 (laureth in the name does not mean sulfate).
4. Detergents that contain the following ingredients are the most natural; however, their effectiveness however is not enough for most consumers to switch: baking soda, soda ash, hydrogen peroxide, and soap from nuts (soap nuts).

What Are Sulfates?

"Sulfates are synthetic ingredients partially based on sulfur, which is derived from petrolatum or other sources," explains Yves Lanctôt, a chemist and product consultant in Laval, Quebec. "However, sulfates are not just petrolatum derived. The largest part of the molecule comes from lauryl alcohol, which is derived from coconut oil or other plants. To make sulfates, lauryl alcohol is reacted with sulfuric acid. Sulfur can be found naturally on earth, but for manufacturing it's generally produced using petrolatum."[7, 8]

FABRIC SOFTENER
AND DRYER SHEETS

Warm, soft, fluffy towels have become a symbol of wholesome goodness and comfort. Unfortunately the liquid softeners that make them fluffy are a major trigger of asthma and may not be what you want to breathe in. Although most are readily biodegradable, they are indeed putting a coating on your clothes, and this coating provides the static-free softness and leaves the strong scent behind, which is inhaled, touches your skin, and in the case of sheets and pillow cases, you are pretty much enveloped in it.

Most brands and certainly all natural ones, use a plant-based derived softener; but like detergents, these are processed. The "quats" or quaternary ammonium compounds[9] used to make fabric softeners are also used in hair conditioners as a softener.

In addition to these quats, silicone is often added to create a coating on the clothing. This coating is what locks in softness and fragrance. It also means it won't wash off as much as a detergent would and is indeed leaving behind a residue. This can make things quite problematic if you suffer from asthma.

Impact on the Environment

They do make dryer sheets out of paper, but my testing has found them to be completely ineffective and simply a waste of money. Nonpaper dryer sheets work, but nonwoven substrate dryer sheets are a polyester and not readily biodegradable.

The most commonly used ingredients for softening in *natural* softeners are dihydrogenated palmoylethyl hydroxyethylmonium methosulfate and dioleoylethyl hydroxyethylmonium methosulfate. They are common fabric softeners and also found in hair conditioners and skin-softening products for shaving. They are considered better than average when it comes to biodegradability but are still found in our waterways. Both are derived from palm oil, which is linked to deforestation and human rights abuse.[10]

In non-natural products, like Downy®, diethyl ester dimethyl ammonium chloride is what is used. It is not derived from anything natural as far as I could find and causes respiratory issues. It is also used as a disinfectant and is antibacterial.

Impact on Your Health

Both of the natural palm oil–based surfactants mentioned do not have respiratory warnings for inhalation. However, the ingredient used to soften in Downy has many links to respiratory concerns. If you have chronic obstructive pulmonary disorder (COPD), asthma, or respiratory concerns, stay away from that product or any other brands that use it. Use a solution or a natural product that is otherwise suggested.

How to Detox

Fabric softener is a product we really don't need. A natural, sulfate-free detergent will not require the use of a fabric softener. I use my detergent and have no need for softener—even for towels. You can avoid static cling by not drying any clothing from man-made materials—polyester, fleece—and letting them hang dry. These generate static and by line drying them, you can avoid softener all together. Vinegar is a natural softener and can be used in your wash. I add one-half cup with my favorite essential oil and do not get a strong residue of vinegar after drying. I have tried the dryer balls—wool and plastic—and have not found them to be helpful, althouogh I know many who love them.

WHITENERS AND OPTICAL BRIGHTENERS

Optical brighteners are not biodegradable and have toxicity concerns. They do not actually whiten or brighten clothing, but they do apply a chemical coating that makes them appear brighter and whiter. There are also potential health concerns for humans, and the EPA recommends manufacturers do not use them or choose ones that are "lower" on the toxicity scale.[11]

Bleach has long been used to whiten whites and disinfect. I will elaborate on this more in cleaning, but the overuse of bleach has been found to cause more respiratory issues, and the germs it is supposed to kill is lowering immune systems and irritating lungs. If you have COPD, asthma, or respiratory issues, do not use bleach and certainly don't use it on your clothing.

Oxy whitener uses peroxide and soda ash, but the real power house in that product is the borax. Borax is a natural substance, and I use it in our Good Home stain remover. If you look up borax, you will find many opposing opinions. We use it in liquid form; however in a powder form one should exercise caution. Don't use it on your skin or inhale the powder. In a liquid form and in the washer, it is perfectly safe and does a good job at removing stains and whitening. It is also mined responsibly in Boron, California.

I have found 20 Mule Borax to be the best solution to whitening and also separating of clothes to be the best solution.

CHAPTER 12

HOME CLEANING

THIS CHAPTER will explore how the need to be clean is causing more harm than good and that the desire to bleach and sanitize everything is making us all unhealthy. To change our cleaning products, we will need to redefine clean. We have become a society that believes cleanliness is healthiness, and this is not true.

A few major concerns are:

- Overuse of bleach lowers your immune system. A 2015 study showed that in homes with heavy use of bleach, the children had a 20 percent higher risk of having the flu at least once in the previous year, a 35 percent higher risk of recurrent tonsillitis, and an 18 percent higher risk for any recurrent infection.[1]
- Increased breathing difficulty for asthma, allergy, chronic obstructive pulmonary disorder (COPD), and other breathing ailments because of high volatile organic compounds (VOCs).[2]
- Decreased resistance to germs, which increases our use of medicines and antibiotics.
- Increased dermatitis for people and pets.
- Exposure to harmful chemicals and known carcinogens.
- Alters our hormone regulation.
- Pollution of our waters, Earth, and fish.

But aren't they tested for safety?

Unless the product is making a claim such as will kill roaches, will kill germs and staph or contains severely toxic ingredients, a product can be put on the shelf without any testing. Most large companies test for efficacy and also for skin and eye irritation on animals (sadly), but long-term hazards to humans are not conducted on everyday cleaning products. In fact, cleaning products are so unregulated, that ingredients do not need to be listed. Anything could be in there—and often it is.

Having spent nearly three decades of my life in this industry, I can tell you that it still has so much work to do. There is little care given to ingredients unless efficacy is involved. Consumers want to kill it, bleach it, and sanitize it, and big cleaning companies are more than happy to meet these requests—but at what cost?

The following are ingredients to avoid and look out for in your cleaning products. From surface cleaners, to dish soaps and glass cleaners, they are chemical filled and could be causing you respiratory issues, skin irritation, and even nausea. Considering we use them daily and they touch our skin and surfaces where we prepare food, we should give them great thought. Most major brands are loaded with chemicals, bleaches, antibacterial agents, and more and are doing you much more harm than good. Many carry huge warnings such as do not swallow, use with ventilation, and skin and eye irritant; yet consumers use these on their kitchen tables, their children's high chairs, their kitchen counters, and places where we eat. What sense does that make?

TETRAPOTASSIUM EDTA

Here is a warning on the MSDS for Tetrapotassium EDTA, which is an ingredient found in many traditional cleaners, including surface cleaners, detergents, and liquid soaps—all going down our drains at rapid rates—its primary function is to remove soap scum and hard scale.

H302 (100%): Harmful if swallowed [Warning: Acute toxicity, oral: Category 4]

H319 (100%): Causes serious eye irritation [Warning: Serious eye damage/eye irritation: Category 2A]

H412 (100%): Harmful to aquatic life with long-lasting effects [Hazardous to the aquatic environment, long-term hazard: Category 3]

ETHANOLAMINE

Another ingredient commonly found is ethanolamine. This ingredients is a solvent and is used in hair dye, dry cleaning, and fracking—yes, fracking and has been considered as a possible scrub for those involved in chemical warfare. It is found in Formula 409 Multisurface cleaner and many others. A toxicity report is available at the following URL, https://pubchem.ncbi.nlm.nih.gov/compound/Ethanolamine#section =Antidote-and-Emergency-.

Toxicity Summary

HUMAN EXPOSURE AND TOXICITY: A concentration of 5.9 percent is irritating to human skin. Symptoms associated with central nervous system depression in humans include increased blood pressure, diuresis, salivation, and pupillary dilation. Large doses produce sedation, coma, and death following depression of blood pressure and cardiac collapse. 2-Aminoethanol inhalation by humans has been reported to cause immediate allergic responses of dyspnea and asthma and clinical symptoms of acute liver damage and chronic hepatitis. ANIMAL STUDIES: Undiluted liquid causes redness and swelling when applied to the skin of the rabbit. Administration of 2-aminoethanol by the intravenous route in dogs produced increased blood pressure, diuresis, salivation, and pupillary dilation. Rats, mice, rabbits, and guinea pigs exposed to vapor or mist at high concentrations (up to 1,250 ppm) developed pulmonary, hepatic, and renal lesions. In a 90-day subacute oral toxicity study of 2-aminoethanol in rats that a maximum daily dose of 0.32 g/kg resulted in no effect; 0.64 g/kg/day resulted in altered liver or kidney wt; and at 1.28 g/kg death occurred. It is considered to be liver toxin. No treatment-related effects were noted in dogs administered as much as 22 mg/kg/d of 2-aminoethanol for 2 years. In developmental studies in rabbits, maternal toxicity was seen at the two higher dose levels (25, 75 mg/kg body weight) as skin irritation and at the highest dose level as reduced weight gain. There was no treatment-related effect on the incidence of any fetal variation or malformation or on the number of malformed fetuses. 2-Aminoethanol has been demonstrated to be non-mutagenic in the Ames Salmonella typhimurium assay, with and without S9 metabolic activation, using TA 1535, TA 1537, TA 1538, TA 98, and TA 100; and also negative in the *Escherichia coli* assay, Saccharomyces gene conversion assay, and rat liver chromosome assay. ECOTOXICITY STUDIES: Aquatic toxicity tests were conducted using zebra fish fry (*Brachydanio rerio*) and the unicellular algae Isochrysis galbana (a flagellate) and *Chaetoceros gracilis* (a diatom). Inhibition of cell division, chlorophyll content, and $(14)CO_2$ uptake in the algae were sensitive end points. 2-Aminoethanol had an LC50 in the zebra fish fry higher than 5,000 mg/L.

DIETHYLENEAMINE PENTA ACETATE (DTPA)

This is used in multisurface cleaners, hair dyes, and also in an emergency for exposure to plutonium, so it makes perfect sense because you should use this daily in your surface cleaner right?

It falls under California's Proposition 65 and is shown to have a "slight" cancer risk according to its MSDS.[3]

2-HEXOXYETHANOL AND BUTOXYPROPANOL

Both are solvents used to help you clean and also used in fracking. Both are irritating to the skin and lungs, with 2-hexoxyethanol being the worse. Butoxypropanol has been shown to be toxic to rats and mice and cause developmental issues, and it may be a human endocrine disruptor. The FDA allows manufacturers to rinse fruits and vegetables with butoxypropanol.

TRICLOSAN

Triclosan is an ingredient that was banned in hand sanitizers, yet the FDA continues to allow it in dish soaps, hand soaps, surface cleaners, and toothpaste. Research has shown that triclosan does the following:

- Alters hormone regulation in animals.
- Might contribute to the development of antibiotic-resistant germs.
- Might be harmful to the immune system.

"When you use a product containing triclosan, you can absorb a small amount through your skin or mouth. A large 2008 study, which was designed to assess exposure to triclosan in a representative sample of U.S. children and adults, found triclosan in the urine of nearly 75 percent of those tested."[4]

Triclosan has shown to be no more effective at killing germs than regular soap and water. Ironic, given that it is being added in dish soap, which is primarily soap and water.

SODIUM DODECYLBENZENESULFONATE

Sodium dodecylbenzenesulfonate is used in popular scrubs and is flammable and carries an inhalation warning.

TRICHLOROCYANURIC ACID

Trichlorocyanuric acid is also popular in scrubs and carries a serious warning.

Signal: Warning

GHS Hazard Statements

Aggregated GHS information from twenty notifications provided by 310 companies to the ECHA C&L Inventory. Each notification may be associated with multiple companies.

H272 (100%): May intensify fire; oxidizer [Warning: Oxidizing liquids; Oxidizing solids: Category 3]

H302 (100%): Harmful if swallowed [Warning: Acute toxicity, oral: Category 4]

H319 (100%): Causes serious eye irritation [Warning: Serious eye damage/eye irritation: Category 2A]

H335 (100%): May cause respiratory irritation [Warning: Specific target organ toxicity, single exposure; Respiratory tract irritation: Category 3]

H400 (99.68%): Very toxic to aquatic life [Warning: Hazardous to the aquatic environment, acute hazard: Category 1]

H410 (100%): Very toxic to aquatic life with long-lasting effects [Warning: Hazardous to the aquatic environment, long-term hazard: Category 1]

Information may vary between notifications depending on impurities, additives, and other factors. The percentage value in parentheses indicates the notified classification ratio from all companies. Only hazard codes with percentage values above 10% are shown.[5]

BLEACH

So many people associate this chemical with clean and that is unfortunate. Bleach is a powerful killer of germs and not something any of us need to use on a daily basis. The addiction is real, and I lost the battle with my own grandmother who added one tablespoon to her dish water every day. Bleach is made by heating saltwater at such a high temperature that it changes composition. It is added to our drinking water and is a powerful disinfectant. It also has been shown in a 2015 study to cause more harm than good when used daily. In fact, homes that use bleach regularly have a higher rate of flus and respiratory illness. The use of it in every single cleaner is lowering people's immune system. I have bleach in my home and use less than a tablespoon every two weeks with a toothbrush to clean grout in my kitchen sink. That is it.

How to Detox

There are nearly fifty multisurface cleaners and dish soaps on the market, and all of them promise you a pure clean house and none of them explaining to you at what cost. No consumer is going to take an hour of research to examine the ingredients unless they already are fully aware of the harms in the products and won't buy them anyhow. My hope is that you do make the switch to a more natural brand. There are many out there that work. These are far better options than regular surface cleaners. I personally use our vinegar and castile soap formulation, which cleans better than any chemical solvent. Vinegar has long been used to deodorize, cut grease, and bring sparkle to glass. The addition of essential oils and castile soap make it a great germ fighter and cleaner and safe to use.

I also promise that by switching your home will not be less clean. In fact, you may notice that you cough less, your air feels cleaner, and you get sick less. In fact give yourself a detox; try three months using natural cleaners or vinegar and water and baking soda. See if you feel healthier and then try a traditional cleaner. I would bet that the fumes will overwhelm you so much in fact, that you will wonder how and why you used such toxic products all these years. If vinegar, water, and baking soda don't appeal to you, try a natural cleaner on the market. These are much better options, although it should be noted that they are still chemicals. My own brand and all the others out there that are 90 percent or more plant derived, but the ingredients from the plants like coconut are very processed and turned into something much different than coconuts and the process, called *ethoxylation*, does add inert chemicals in the process. Look for sulfate-free options, which will be the most gentle and are much better alternatives to the harsh and harmful ingredients found in the regular brands and will also bring a middle ground to an industry much in need of "cleaning up."

CHAPTER 13

SPECIALTY CLEANERS

Natural Recipes for Stain Removers, Rug Cleaners, and Metal Cleaners

METAL POLISHES and stain removers are often the most toxic of the bunch and carry hefty warnings and for good reason. Filled with VOCs and solvents, they harm our environment and our bodies in an effort to make things "clean." Here are some natural remedies to try instead of the toxic standbys.

SILVER POLISH

The warnings on a small tube of metal polish make you question why it was ever invented, let alone why you would use it on your silver and copper cookware that you eat and drink off of. To clean silver, try a solution of cornstarch and water and an old cotton rag. Apply a paste of cornstarch and water to the silver and let it dry, then rub off with a mildly abrasive cloth.

COPPER CLEANER

I have a bright coppered kettle on my stove, and it is one of my favorite things. It tarnishes frequently, and I battled with how to polish it and also still use it without fear of harming my family from the metal polish residue. My son, a lover of science, brought me this great recipe that works like a charm. Using table salt and a scrubber (one specifically that you keep for this use), make a paste with white vinegar and scrub away. The chemical reaction shines copper to a sparkling finish. You can also try this trick with a penny. Wear gloves because both the salt and vinegar are irritating to the skin.

STAIN AND ODOR REMOVER

The best stain and odor remover I have ever found is 20 Mule Team Borax®. This will take out new and old stains and also remove odors from clothing and towels. This is the powerful ingredient in my tried-and-true stain remover and many other natural stain removers. As covered previously, I do not think Borax should be labeled as poorly as the Environmental Working Group has done. Unless it is ingested, there is no harm in using this product to clean. This is why when looking at ingredients you have to look at everything individually and cannot create a computer algorithm because you simply will not get honest results. I use a cup of this once a month in my washer to deodorize it, and it can also be added with soap when washing towels and workout gear to deodorize. To clean a stain on any fabric that can tolerate soap and water, make a paste using a tablespoon of borax with one-half teaspoon of liquid castile soap (Dr. Bronner's is a good brand) and a little water. Scrub the stain with a designated tooth brush or other scrubber used just for that purpose. Wash or wipe with clear water. You can also make a spray solution in a glass bottle and use this for rug stains. Just add enough water to the recipe to make it sprayable. It works wonderfully on old stains too.

AIR FRESHENER

When you spray regular store-brand air fresheners, you are not cleaning the air, and further, only causing harm to your respiratory system. You can easily make your own and save money while you are at it. Simply add ten drops of your favorite essential oil—I like grapefruit or lemon or balsam fir as an air freshener—to an eight-ounce glass sprayer bottle purchased for this use. Fill three-quarters to the top with water and then add one-quarter witch hazel. This is safe to use and does the trick. The witch hazel works as a preservative and is not as overwhelming as alcohol, which is in most air fresheners.

CARPET FRESHENER

The sprinkling of powders does far more harm than good. Powders not only harm your vacuum motor over time, but they also are never fully removed from the carpet, staying in the fibers where your children and pets roll around on. To add scent to the air while you vacuum, add a few tablespoons of dried lavender flowers to your vacuum bag. Every time you turn it on, your vacuum will smell wonderful.

WOOD CONDITIONER

Regular dusting is all I do for my wood furniture, refraining from polish. However for my kitchen cutting block, which can dry out with so much use, I condition it using coconut oil. I would never put mineral oil—food grade or not—on my cutting board, where I cut my organic veggies and fruits. It makes no sense to me. Mineral oil is pure petroleum and not meant to be ingested. Instead I use a little coconut oil. It is safe, effective, and does not go rancid or get sticky like some cooking oils do. And I have zero concerns about it touching my food.

DRAIN CLEANER

A little bit of baking soda and some vinegar down the drain will deodorize and also amuse your little ones with a mini volcano. Although it may decrease grease in the pipes, you should make it a practice to never pour grease down the drain. All liquid and solid fats should be poured into a container like a soup can and then thrown away in the garbage.

STAINLESS STEEL POLISHER

First clean your fridge or oven or appliances with a vinegar and water solution. Once dry, add a dab of olive oil to a dry cloth and rub onto the stainless steel in circular motions.

PART IV

DETOX YOUR
WARDROBE

I T WAS QUITE a surprise to me to find that our desire for immediate, inexpensive clothing is one of the largest sources of environmental pollution and human rights violations. I personally never gave it a second thought until a friend, who also happens to be a fashion designer, suggested I watch *The True Cost*.[1] It is a wonderful documentary that reveals the "true costs" of our need for cheap, inexpensive clothing.

This is not just a manufacturing issue but a socioeconomic one. The need for inexpensive clothing in the United States is real. As of 2015, 2.6 million people in the workforce earned an hourly wage of $7.25 or less. That is $290 a week—gross—before taxes are taken out.[2] Certainly not enough to pay $75 for one item of clothing that is ethically made, with organic cotton and natural dyes. The need for $10 dresses at Old Navy is understandable, but shopping at fast-fashion stores—like Old Navy®, Forever 21®, Zara®, the Gap®, lululemon®—to get a whole bunch of clothes for a cheap price that you wear just once and it either falls apart or shrinks is causing massive pollution. The cheap clothing we so easily throw out or donate after wearing three times has a very dirty secret. The fact is people don't want our cheap clothing in the United States or abroad, and we are paying—by the boatload—to dump our cheap finds in Third-World countries—where we pollute their land with our trash. Or as in East Africa, we put local clothing artisans out of business because the "donated" clothes are sold, and locals stop buying from their communities' dressmakers.

In chapter 14, we will delve into this and learn what we can do and what is being done to make fashion more sustainable. We will also look at the hidden toxins in clothing—from dry cleaning to plastic shoes to lead in necklaces and fire retardants in our kid's pajamas.

What can we do to make sure we are not inadvertently hurting ourselves or our planet with our innocent choices?

CHAPTER 14

FAST FASHION

WHAT IS fast fashion? Like food, we get clothing, shoes, jewelry, and bags quickly and cheaply. Our options are endless with racks upon racks of new clothing in the stores every week—sometimes even twice a week. And not just in one color, but maybe in three or even five or eight colors.

Nearly every piece of new clothing available in stores for purchase was made outside of the United States and manufactured with harm to the person who made it, to the local land and water, and to the overall health of our planet. And even if it was made in the United States, there is a good chance it was produced by an undocumented immigrant who is not being paid legal wage—far from it in fact.[1]

I could not find one major clothing line that could show sustainable and ethical production. Not one. Even companies like Patagonia—who truly stand behind ethical fashion—are hard pressed to say their manufacturers are 100 percent paying fair wages and not employing children. The model of fashion simply does not allow it. Everything must be faster and cheaper, and someone is going to take the hit—that is usually the worker who most likely can't read or write and is easily fired.

So what is the true cost of that five-dollar shirt you just bought?

FABRIC

It takes 2,700 liters of water to make one (nonorganic) cotton shirt—from the growing of the cotton to the manufacturing of it. Cotton takes up slightly more than 2 percent of all land used for agriculture, but it accounts for 24 percent of global pesticide use, which makes it the most pesticide-intensive crop.[2]

DYES

Clothing dyes and the pretreatment of the cloth before it is dyed constitute 20 percent of worldwide water pollution. The majority of our clothing is made in China or India where the laws are minimal on corporate pollution. The dyes are frequently dumped—chemicals and all—into the seas. Per China Water Watch,[3] it is estimated that 70 percent of lakes and rivers in China are polluted, as well as 90 percent of the groundwater. In all, an estimated 320 million Chinese do not have access to clean drinking water—more than the entire population of the United States. Ironically, the United States is the biggest contributor to the purchasing of the Chinese-made clothing, taking 75 percent of what China produces, but then more than 65 percent of the world's clothing is made in China.

LABOR

From child labor to women hiding their pregnancies in fear of being fired (pregnant women are seen as slower), this is one industry that needs to do a deep dive into their ethics. Child workers are prized for their small hands and skills and often used to sew intricate details like sequins and embroidery. I searched and searched and could not find one clothing manufacturer who could claim zero human rights violations—including manufacturers in the United States. The fact is you cannot sell a shirt for five dollars and expect everyone to be paid a living wage. Although companies are putting rules into place and have their "ethics" posted on their website, unless they own the factories and hold employees accountable, the layers for corruption are immense and hard to control. From inspectors being paid off to falsify reports, to workers being killed by the police for protesting, fashion is one of the worst businesses out there when it comes to treatment of humans.[4]

WHEN YOU ARE DONE WEARING IT

So you wore the blue shirt a few times and it lost its color or doesn't fit right. Where does it go next? Even mass clothing resellers like Buffalo Exchange won't take an Old Navy piece, so you bag it up and donate it to Goodwill. Taking a tax deduction and leaving happy and feeling like you are helping the world with your donation. Sadly, even the Goodwill doesn't want your fast fashion. Goodwill has higher specifications than this cheap, disposable clothing, so they pass it on to a clothing warehouse who distributes the unwanted shirt. After sifting through the items for any "finds" like vintage jeans that were missed—the stuff they can't sell to Japan (vintage) or Eastern Europe (cold weather gear) —gets shipped off to Africa. In the 1980s, Africa dropped their policies to protect local businesses, so secondhand clothing is welcomed there. And surprise! In the1990s, African textile companies spiraled down and went out of business because of it. By 2004, 81 percent of clothing purchased in Uganda was secondhand, and in 2005, nearly 25 percent of it was deemed unsellable because of poor quality.[5]

Let's say the five-dollar blue shirt is deemed unusable for resell, what's next? It is then shredded for rags and insulation, and even the rags eventually make their way to the landfill—where they sit in heaps—producing methane that pollutes our climate even further.

And that is just one five-dollar shirt; 13 million tons of clothing is thrown out every year in the United States alone. Americans trash 85 percent of their wardrobe every year.[6]

An article by Alden Wicker for *Newsweek* was one of the most comprehensive I have seen on what happens to our clothing; I highly recommend you read its entirety.[7]

What can we do? This is coming to a crisis and all big fast-fashion companies know it. There are efforts from retailers like H&M to pay you for your old H&M clothing or offer a discount, but honestly most of this is just marketing right now. Unless we get the majority of our thrown-out clothing to be repurposed or truly recycled, it does not solve the problem. The secondhand clothing industry is coming to a point where they cannot handle the amount of clothing that is coming in. There is no place for it to go but the landfill. And with stores changing their inventory with new items as quick as two times a week, the pipelines are flowing with more clothing, not less. Like nearly everything reported in this book, it is going to come down to the businesses manufacturing the clothing to make the changes and invest a significant amount of their earnings to figuring out how to solve this problem, or we will literally be buried in it.

What can we do?

REPURPOSE

I had the opportunity to visit the New York headquarters of Eileen Fisher, whose owner by the same name is actively seeking ways to make a difference. Fisher sees the writing on the wall and is taking responsibility for her company's part in this industry. They have a separate department dedicated to finding ways to make their clothing process have as minimal of an impact as possible. Last summer I visited a "pop-up store" they had in Brooklyn featuring their "greeneileen" (www.greeneileen.org) repurposed brand, which takes old Eileen Fisher clothing and gives it a new life and a new design. I also had the opportunity to meet some of the graduates on the design team—a group of young women whose ethics and efforts were true. They will be the first to admit that this task will need the entire industry to come together if efforts are to be made.

RECYCLING

Ideally, we would love to recycle our clothing, right? Unfortunately, the chemicals and dyes used to make most of our clothing gives off toxic gases when burned or incinerated. Polyester is a petroleum product, so it would serve us well to recycle it for many reasons. Incineration and recycling are tricky. You cannot mix fibers and the fibers need to be separated and of a high quality. Low-quality fibers simply shred and do not make good thread. But there are companies out there who are working hard to improve this. One such company, Dutch Awearness,[8] is able to recycle work uniforms—such as flight attendants jackets—into new clothing. Patagonia (another company taking ownership of it's part in industry waste) has invested in the recycling of their polyester fleece products and have a few available online.

BUY

Ultimately we need to buy less. I love to shop, but after watching the film *The True Cost*, my shopping has probably decreased by 90 percent. Now when I purchase I try to buy a piece that may cost more, but will also last for three years. So much is bought on impulse. If you see something you "have to have," give yourself twenty-four hours to think about it. If you wake up in the morning and still want it, then buy it. But chances are, the desire will have left.

We also need to repurpose our clothes. Look for ways to turn your old items into something new. Or shop at secondhand retailers. What was once a trend for me in high school is back again as I approach fifty! Many of my friends and my mom's friends shop second-hand stores for new pieces. It just makes sense.

If you have one kid like I do, hand down your clothes to friends. Kids' rapid growth ensures the need for new clothes every six months. We offset this by handing ours down to friends with younger kids.

When you buy new, look for items that are organic cotton and wool. Organic cotton does not use the pesticides that nonorganic cotton does. Try to buy clothing that is handmade. Etsy and flea markets are great resources to find new designers and support their work. I used to think buying clothing made in the United States made a difference, but that is not the case. Human rights abuses happen here just as they do anywhere. They happen less because we do not manufacture as much here now. If you buy polar fleece or other petroleum, polyester, man-made fabrics, buy from a company like Patagonia who is putting their money into making this industry more sustainable.

And lastly, shop your own closet. Take the time to go through and find the things you didn't know you had. Or have a clothing trade with friends. As they say, someone's trash is someone else's treasure.

CHAPTER 15

HIDDEN TOXINS IN OUR WARDROBES

THIS CHAPTER covers some of the things you don't even think about carrying toxins—like shoes or your kids' paja-mas. I know personally I never even gave it a second thought to let my son wear plastic shoes before I even considered the BPAs.

As I have found while writing this book, nothing is safe. Our government has given the safety reigns over to the businesses, and they are far more concerned in getting you a new product as quickly and cheaply as possible. Safety and research are rarely a consideration.

This chapter will take a look at those random items that we don't think twice about but that can carry a lot of damage without us even realizing it.

JEWELRY

We all have heard the concerns of lead in cheap kids jewelry from China, but I always thought of that to be in the paint. Unfortunately it is in the metal, too. While looking at lead, I came across a valuable human resource, Tamara Rubin (http://tamararubin.com/mislead/) whose own children were poisoned by lead from the repainting of their house. Tamara's children innocently played outside while the contractors scraped away old lead paint and ensured her they were doing it safely. She has turned her pain into a crusade to help us all understand that lead is not an issue in the 1970s, but alive and well in the twenty-first century. After watching her film *MisLead*, I wondered of course about my own items. I have many antique jewelry pieces that I cherish and wear, but they are not pure gold or silver. Most antique jewelry is not. Well of course after doing a simple swab test from a kit I got on Amazon, I had several pieces that I had to stop wearing because of the lead content.

New jewelry—that may be gold or silver plated or stainless steel—often has lead in it. Mine sure did. I have a "metal" bracelet that tested positive for lead, and I paid twenty-five dollars for it! Of course, it wasn't marked because as I said in the beginning of this chapter, your safety is not the manufacturer's number-one concern—fast and cheap is. If you needed an excuse to buy pure gold or silver or platinum jewelry, this is it. Even some of my copper wrapped wire necklaces were not pure. A medallion purchased from two monks in support of their monastery that I treasure, tested positive for lead when I thought it was brass.

Too much lead in adults causes headaches and stomach issues, but for kids it is much worse. Particularly when younger, they are far more susceptible to the damages of lead's poison. Many children who have ADHD often test positive for lead poisoning, but doctors rarely test for it anymore. Unless you are living on public assistance or in Section 8 housing where lead paint is still on the walls, they do not think it is an issue for you, when in fact it is. If you are renovating an old house or live in one, the old paint on the porch or the wood door that was stripped could have enormously high amounts of lead in it. The cheap costume jewelry you let your kids wear during dress up or the bracelet your baby puts in his mouth can be filled with lead.

Even the charms on new shoes have lead, actually killing a young child who accidentally swallowed them.[1]

There are simple swab kits you can purchase on Amazon or at a hardware store to test your jewelry and I would recommend you do—particularly items that are painted a bright color or not a certified precious metal. Anything that has been painted or glazed or is a nonprecious metal can contain lead—even if they are beautiful or fun. Cheap plastic Mardi Gras beads, for instance, have high lead content in them. If you have young children, keep the fake jewelry off them and certainly away from any toddlers who still put stuff in their mouths.

You can make cute things from wood beads, cloth, shells, feathers, and other natural items.

PLASTIC SHOES AND SHOE DYES

From ages four to seven, my son must have worn plastic shoes nearly every single day. They are easy to slip on, lightweight, and don't stay wet. I never even thought twice about my son's shoes having BPAs and leaching harmful endocrine-disrupting chemicals into his body via his sweaty sockless feet in those shoes. I shouldn't have had to if manufacturers were doing the right thing. Of course, then I realize I have been wearing plastic shoes all my life, too—we just called them flip flops. Plastic shoes contain all sorts of BPAs and phthalates and chemicals just like the bottles do. Except you are wearing them—without socks—on moist sweaty feet, which makes them the perfect vessel to leak into your body.[2] Safer options would include fabric soles—but make sure they are dye free. My son's feet turned red from the dyes on his $100 Birkenstocks. Dyes contain all sorts of chemicals, including chromium and mercury, and the leather dye business is a dirty one. Many countries where we get our cheap leather from do not participate in clean manufacturing processes—just like clothing—and the dyes go into the water and onto your feet. The workers doing the dying suffer the most. In the summer or when you go sockless, choose flip flops that have leather soles that are natural in color and dye free and pick a high-quality sandal—not the cheap plastic ones. If you must have plastic, look at the Native brand, who states on their website that their shoes are free of BPAs and phthalates.[3]

FLAME-RETARDANT CLOTHING

A friend and colleague, Jon Wheelan, who produced and directed the movie *Stink*, had his daughters pajamas tested for chemicals when he noticed they smelled and also had been treated with something. He called the company who manufactured them and got no answer, so he tested them himself and what he found was awful.

Flame retardants were developed by cigarette manufacturers because smokers were dying falling asleep with their cigarettes in the

1970s—when 40 percent of people smoked. The government urged manufacturers to create safer cigarettes but instead they teamed up with chemical suppliers to create a product that our furniture, clothing, and mattresses are doused with. Flame-retardant chemicals are found in all of our blood. They contain harmful chemicals that we breath in every time we lay on our mattress or sit on a couch treated with them. Some chemicals were such harmful neurotoxins they were banned, but of course, are still found in flame retardants to this day because no one checks and the chemical itself was not banned. Two articles—one from Yale University and one from the *New York Times*—unveil the harms of this archaic product.[4, 5] I suggest you read them, be aware, and make sure you purchase clothing and furniture that were not treated, if you can.

DRY CLEANING

As a rule, I avoid the dry cleaners as much as possible, preferring to hand wash what I can. This is not entirely possible because I have good sweaters that hand washing simply does not treat well. Many of my good cashmere sweaters have lost their shape from hand washing, and I have a few silk tops with pleats that would fall apart even with the gentlest of hand washing. So although it may be no more than three times a year, I do make it to the dry cleaners. I have noticed the term *organic* and *green* dry cleaning around the city, but my clothes still come back smelling like chemicals. Looking into this further, many customers are feeling they have a safe option, but what they are getting is a "safer" option—there is a difference. Although cleaners throw around the terms *green* and *organic*, they are not regulated by the government, so they can call it whatever they wish, misleading us all to think this is a healthy way to clean our clothes.

There are three options out there; two are chemical solvents and one uses carbon dioxide. An article from the *New York Sun* explained the processes well:

> GreenEarth Cleaning is a process that involves a nontoxic, chemically inert, silicone-based chemical solvent. When disposed of, its ingredients decompose within days into silica, water, and trace amounts of carbon dioxide. All studies, including independent evaluations, have deemed it harmless to handlers and the environment.

Hydrocarbon is the oldest and cheapest alternative to perc. It uses a volatile, carbon-based compound, similar to perc in chemical composition. Largely manufactured by ExxonMobil, the solvent is less hazardous to workers and the environment than perc, but can also result in a strange odor on clothing. "A lot of people don't like how it can leave a smell," the owner of Casa Organic Dry Cleaners in New York, Ruben Sadykov, said. "But it depends on what needs to be cleaned. Sometimes it works best."

CO_2 cleaning is the newest and priciest technology. It involves using special equipment to convert carbon dioxide from gas to liquid, which is then used to clean the clothes. After that, the carbon dioxide is converted back into gas and released. It is viewed as environmentally friendly and, in addition to the process of wet cleaning, the best for keeping fabric chemical-free.[6]

Perchloroethylene (perc), which is the solvent used in traditional dry cleaning, was found by the EPA likely to be a carcinogen when inhaled. This means that when you bring home dry cleaning that was traditionally cleaned and you unwrap it, you are inhaling a carcinogen. This also means every time you wear the piece of clothing, you are inhaling carcinogens.

The options here are better, but not without chemicals. GreenEarth Cleaning uses a chemical called D5, which has been shown to cause stomach cancer in mice. Other "green options" use a chemical called DF-2000; produced by Exxon mobile, it is classified as a neurotoxin by the EPA.

If you have to dry clean, find a carbon-dioxide cleaner or ask if "wet cleaning" is available. It uses dipropylene glycol as a solvent in its process that is much less toxic than the others. It is not chemical free, but it is much better.

Always take the clothing out of the plastic right away and air it out—outside if you can—or you are just releasing the chemicals in your air at home.

PESTICIDES IN WOOL

How is this natural fiber toxic? Industrialized wool is no different than farming and sheep are often put in inhumane conditions. Sheep are "dipped" in toxic pesticides called OP, which is a nerve gas developed in World War II to prevent the spreading of diseases. Many sheep farmers have suffered from severe illnesses—even died—because of exposure to these pesticides. It is well known in the industry, but it is not something they advertise. Sian Anna Lewis's article from the New Zealand government covers it quite well and does not sugarcoat it.[7]

Dipping is not only harmful to the farmers but also to their land. The practice of dipping often involves a giant puddle or hole in the ground of which a sheep is made to walk a plank to fall into the dip and then pulled out. Sheep can drown in the pesticide or swallow it and die later. The other option is showering, where sheep are sprayed and drenched with pesticide and then made to drip and drain for twenty-four hours and given only water. It is not pleasant and not humane. There are two articles that I found that are targeted to the farmers, explaining the process and also how to protect yourself from the pesticides.[8, 9]

Both traditional and organic wool require a significant amount of water and deplete natural resources in their processing from clippings to yarn.[10] If organic, the sheep may have not been exposed to pesticides, but the washing of the clippings often uses detergents and chemicals that are not friendly to our aquatic system—such as alkylphenol ethoxylates, which are endocrine disruptors and also found in our detergents, cleaning products, pesticides, and automotive products—and get dumped into our waters. When it comes to wool—like food—just buying organic isn't enough. Know your source and ask questions about the entire process, including how they clean it.

PART V

DETOX YOUR STUFF

WE HAVE covered food, water, personal care and cleaning products, our clothing, and what we cook with. But yet there is still so much more. The next three chapters will touch on the many other items we use daily—our phones, our furniture, and the toys our children play with. Although I could write an entire book on furniture alone, these chapters will hopefully bring awareness to a few of the significant issues, so you can make the healthiest choices for you and your family.

First up is a look at the electronics we use. Many of us have been suspect of our devices, and if anything, would like a clear picture of what harms they cause. I think we all are hoping that our cell phone won't turn out to be the cigarette of the twenty-first century. I have a dear friend whose forty-six-year-old husband had colon cancer. The tumor was found in the same spot where he used to wear his blackberry strapped to his hip every single morning—all day long. I wonder how many of these stories are out there and although I am not saying his phone caused this, I would certainly like proof that it didn't. Even after a study came out that young children should not use cell phones next to their heads, I see kids using the phones all the time. Unless we see danger immediately with our own eyes, most of us do not heed the advice of experts such as the American Academy of Pediatrics and continue to use the devices without any concern for future health crisis.

Another product we would expect to be perfectly safe are our children's toys and art supplies. We shouldn't have to think twice, but so many of their toys are made from plastic or contain lead-based inks that are constantly being recalled, yet the few that do get mentioned are just a drop in the bucket. How many are not being tested? Most of the recalls are found by parents doing their due diligence, or in the worst case, after a trip to the hospital. I cringe every time my son wants to put on a removable tattoo or buy a fidget spinner—a recent fad—that may or may not have a high amount of lead. How about all the times we put on face paint for Halloween, only to find it was recalled for lead. Call me crazy, but shouldn't those most at risk for poisoning be the ones we protect? Buying a toy—or anything for that matter—shouldn't be a game of roulette with our health. Don't we want to make sure that our young children are given a healthy start and not have their IQs compromised because there were not enough people checking the new toys coming in from overseas? Why is our government looking to build jobs in industries like coal that pollute our world when so many more jobs are needed to police these pollutants? Chapter 17 will look at this, and hopefully help you in making the safe choice for your family.

Chapter 18 will look at our furniture, paint, and mattresses and uncover the toxins that are automatically put in without us even knowing. Flame retardants, lead, volatile organic compounds, and environmental concerns are all a part of the furniture-manufacturing industry. This final chapter will look at what precautionary measures we should take before buying our next couch.

CHAPTER 16

ELECTRONICS AND CELL PHONES

ELECTROMAGNETIC frequencies (EMF) have come into our lives quickly and without much regulation. EMFs are around us everywhere and you would be hard pressed to escape them, even in the middle of nowhere. Cell towers, Wi-Fi routers, cell phones, cordless phones, tablets, and anything electric emits EMFs. They are designated into three categories

- Extremely low frequency (ELF) items, such as refrigerators, toasters, and other electric appliances.
- Radio frequency (RF) refers to cordless phones and cellular phones.
- "Dirty Electricity" radio frequencies emitted from poor wiring (i.e., high-frequency signals flowing through overloaded wires).

Electricity and the pollution it emits has long been a concern. Women in Long Island were studied for their proximity to EMFs and also pesticide exposure for the unusually high breast cancer incidents in their neighborhood.[1]

So far, there is no conclusive evidence, pointing either way. One study said that high cell phone use increases your risk for cancer,[2] and another says no.[3] The World Health Organization (WHO) is conducting their own study, which has yet to be published because it needs a thorough review.[4]

Given the amount of EMFs we are exposed to daily, we should all demand complete and comprehensive studies be performed. I know I have said this probably in every chapter, but the way of our current world is to put product before health, and unless we demand it, the manufacturers will just do minimal or no testing. In twenty years, we could very well find out that the devices we use are harmful to our health—just like cigarettes.

With new devices coming out every quarter, faster and more powerful, we have gone from 1G to 4G in just a few years, without any studies being done on the increase of this power. A report from U.S. Government Accountability Office recommends the Federal Communications Commission reassess mobile phone safety because the dramatic increase in power and exposure to RFs.[5] The report states,

> The FCC should formally reassess and, if appropriate, change its current RF energy exposure limit and mobile phone testing requirements related to likely usage configurations, particularly when phones are held against the body. FCC noted that a draft document currently under consideration by FCC has the potential to address GAO's recommendations.

For this book, I had the pleasure of corresponding with Dr. Anthony Miller, M.D.[6] Dr. Miller is one of just a handful of experts who work tirelessly in documenting, reporting, and demanding our governments and industries warn the public and do the work to ensure the public's safety. He kindly answered a few of my questions, and I suggest you take a deep dive into his work, which can be found at www.ehtrust.org.

Q: Most people are completely unaware of any concerns regarding electronic devices. They wouldn't even know where to start. In your research and findings, which electronics are the most detrimental to our health? And is it the same for adults as it is children? For instance, I read that cordless phones emit far more EMFs than a cell phone.

A: All devices that depend on Wi-Fi (radio frequency fields [RFF]) if used near a person will potentially adversely affect health—electro-hypersensitivity in those who become sensitive to RFF, and cancer, especially brain and salivary gland cancers in the case of cell phones, but also breast cancer in women who keep cell phones in their bras, and infertility in men and possibly women. These devices include iPads, laptop computers, Wi-Fi-linked baby alarms, house monitors as well as cell phones. The access points for Wi-Fi in homes and schools, smart meters and cell towers also emit RFF. For all emitters of RFF, the closer to humans the greater the exposure; this is why we say "Distance is your friend." As cell phones tend to be used and kept very close to the body, these are probably the most dangerous for human health.

The adverse effects of RFF are likely to be much greater in children than in adults, though for cancer, this will not necessarily increase the risk of cancer in childhood, but in adult life, as cancer has a long natural history.

The studies that have been done (in Sweden) comparing the adverse effects of cordless phones and cell phones suggest that both are equally dangerous in increasing the risk of brain cancer.

Q: What can we do to protect ourselves from the Wi-Fi that surrounds us everywhere from our homes to our work to our schools?

A: Reduce usage as much as possible, keep cell phones away from the body, use hands-free devices rather than keep the cell phone close to the ear, turn off all sources of RFF at night (use timed electricity control switches), connect computers to the Internet using wired (Ethernet) connections rather than Wi-Fi. We should adopt the principle that years ago we learnt to apply to exposure to ionizing radiation (X-rays, etc.), keep the dose *As Low as Reasonably Achievable* (the *ALARA* principle). Another term used is to adopt the precautionary principle, remembering that if we fail to take action now, and allow exposures to RFF to accumulate, when absolute proof of the dangers is available it will be too late to prevent a public health disaster.

Q: Why in your opinion are these devices so unregulated? What can we do to protect ourselves from being essentially experimented on? Where can we get involved to make a difference?

A: The problem is that for the majority of people, devices powered by Wi-Fi have become an essential part of life. This coupled with their ready availability have convinced the majority that there can be no hazard. It is difficult to overcome this belief as absolute proof of harm is demanded, which in the early years of human exposure to a potential hazard cannot be expected. To overcome this we have to use every opportunity to urge those in charge of the organizations meant to protect us, school boards, governments at all levels, international agencies such as the World Health Organization, to accept there are potential dangers and adopt the precautionary principle and take appropriate action. We are faced with many deniers, often supported by industry, who refuse to even consider the possibility of a hazard.

Q: It came out recently that cell phones increase cancer tumors in the brain—yet no one has stopped reducing their use. People still give them to their children. I personally do not let my son talk on the phone or use it in Wi-Fi mode. But it is extremely difficult when new games requiring Wi-Fi like *Pokémon Go* come out. Ultimately it is the responsibility of the parent—but will the government or cell phone manufacturers ever help us and create something safer?

A: The cell phone manufacturers do recognize that there is a potential danger—and that they could face substantial liability law suits in the future. They include warnings in their leaflets about keeping cell phones away from the ear but tend to hide them in small print or inaccessible websites. It is governments who carry the heaviest responsibility to warn the public. We should not let children play with or use devices that depend on RFF.

Q: What safety products do you recommend? Does copper in fact deter EMFs from a cell phone tower or Wi-Fi in your home?

A: There are RF shields that you can purchase—e.g., for installing in walls or near smart meters. I do not know if copper is protective—as it is a good conductor of electricity I suspect not.

Q: Please add anything else you would like to be included on this topic.

A: In 2011, a working group of the International Agency for Research on Cancer, the cancer research wing of the World Health Organization, designated radio frequency fields a category 2B carcinogen, a *possible* human carcinogen. Since that review a number of additional studies have been reported. One of the most important was a large case-control study in France, which found a doubling of risk of glioma, the most malignant form of brain cancer, after two years of exposure to cell phones. After five years exposure the risk was five-fold. They also found that in those who lived in urban environments the risk was even higher. In my view, and that of several of my colleagues, these studies provide evidence that radio frequency fields are not just a *possible* human carcinogen but a *probable* human carcinogen (i.e., IARC category 2A). It would be impossible to ignore such an assessment in regulatory approaches.

It is important to recognize that there are no safe levels of exposure to human carcinogens. Risk increases with increasing intensity of exposure, and for many carcinogens, such as tobacco smoke, even more with increasing duration of exposure. Thus, the only way to avoid the carcinogenic risk is to avoid exposure altogether. This is why we ban known carcinogens from the environment and why much effort is taken to get people, particularly young people, not to smoke. We now recognize that exposure to carcinogens in childhood can increase the risk of cancer in adulthood many years later. Further, people vary in their genetic makeup, and certain genes can make some people more susceptible than others to the effect of carcinogens. It is the young and those who are susceptible that safety codes should be designed to protect

Given my history of breast cancer, I wanted to make sure my new home was electronically safe and called in the services of Matthew Waletzke, Certified Building Biology Environmental Consultant (BBEC) and owner of Healthy Dwellings, a service in New York City and Connecticut that comes and measures the RF wave levels in your home.

My primary concern was the cell tower on top of our roof. My condominium had a sponsor who sold the rights to our roof for his own

Table 16.1

Radio Frequency

This pertains to all forms of wireless transmission originating from both outside and inside the home. These include, but are not limited to cellular phones, Wi-Fi, radio, television, cordless phones, etc. Health effects that have been reported from RF exposure range from headaches and insomnia to altered white blood cells and certain types of cancer. Below are the radio frequencies measured inside the home. Any changes to internal sources are noted in the table.

Location	Radio Frequency "full" Signal in μW/m²
Rooftop (East edge of building in front of access door)	160,000
Apartment PH2 (Living Room)	7,850–20,000
Apartment PH1 (Second-floor Bedroom)	6,480
Apartment PH1 (Living Room)	18,240
PH-level Hallway	230–5,730
Apartment #B (Dining Room)	1,300
Apartment #B (Living Room)	5,900
Apartment #B (Living Room, Verizon router turned off)	1,270
Apartment #B (Master Bedroom)	700
Apartment #B (Bedroom #2)	4,000
Apartment #B (Bedroom #2 with cordless telephone off)	1,150

Equipment used:
Analyzer: Gigahertz Solutions HFE59B Radio Frequency Analyzer
Antenna: Gigahertz Solutions UBB27, broadband, omni-directional 27MHz – 3.3 GHz
Internal exposure guidelines Radio Frequency Radiation (High Frequency, electromagnetic waves):

Location	Limit Based On	Radio Frequency "full" Signal in μW/m²
Canada/USA	Thermal/Heating	10,000,000
Russia/China/Italy/ Most of Eastern Europe	Biological	100,000
Bio-Initiative Report 2007	Biological/Precautionary	1,000
Building Biology Guidelines for Sleeping areas— Germany	Biological/Precautionary	0.1
Average Residential Indoor Exposure	Healthy Dwellings	150–5,000

Values apply to single RF sources (e.g. GSM, UMTS, WiMAX, TETRA, Radio, Television, DECT cordless phone technology, WLAN, etc.) and refer to peak measurements. They do not apply to radar signals.

More critical RF sources like pulsed or periodic signals (mobile phone technology, DECT, WLAN, digital broadcasting, etc.) should be assessed more seriously, especially in the higher ranges, and less critical RF sources like nonpulsed and nonperiodic signals (FM, short, medium, long wave, analog broadcasting, etc.) would be assessed more generously especially in the lower ranges.

profit—with no care for our health—to Verizon. We have more than nine panels on our roof emitting RFs constantly.

As Matthew explained to me, the waves bounce, so although it is on the roof, they can hit a building next to it and then bounce back into my windows. Given the condensed nature of this city, I had no idea what to expect. Cell phone towers on roofs are everywhere—with customers demanding more service, Verizon and landlords are happy to respond. None of us give it any thought, except when we live next door to one.

As Matthew explained to me and as Dr. Miller pointed out, our cordless phones have been emitting high RFs for some time now. In fact, in my apartment report (see Table 16.1), my son's bedroom had a high amount of frequencies because the cordless phone was sitting on my desk next to his bedroom. After we disconnected it, they were reduced significantly.

As you can also see, my fifth-floor apartment, which is two floors below the cell towers, had much less RFs than the penthouse apartments. The highest source of RF waves were from our wireless router, which sits in the living room. The huge source of RF waves in the penthouse—eighteen thousand to be exact—were not from the cell tower, but from the Sonos machine.

What does it all mean? I asked Matthew and here is what he shared with me. The concern with RFs is not the short term but long term. We simply do not know what this is doing to our bodies yet. We do know that those sensitive to RF waves experience sleeplessness and headaches, and most of us instinctively turn off our devices at night. Many of us are addicted to our devices and the ease they bring us, without even realizing our sleepless nights and headaches could be blamed on these nighttime addictions.

WHAT CAN YOU DO?

Personally, I removed all cordless phones in my home and switched to regular dial up. And if I need to walk around, I use a headset on my cell phone. Matthew also explained to me this is a safer option than the cordless phone on my head.

Next, the Wi-Fi router will stay in our living room. It is far from our bedrooms, so I do not turn it off at night. However if it were close by, it would be turned off. This is as simple as flipping a switch.

No Wi-Fi in the bedroom during bedtime. We don't have and will not have a Sonos or other "smart" home devices. My son uses the cell phone on speaker and is not allowed to "hotspot." No playing iPad or iPhone games with the Wi-Fi on. I do not wear or put cell phones or wireless devices on my body.

See if your kids' school is on Wi-Fi. I did, and fortunately there was no Wi-Fi at the time of writing this. If there is Wi-Fi, see what protections are in place and where the routers are placed. Make sure they are safe.

This is a subject I urge you to take seriously and at least limit the use of these Wi-Fi devices in your home. We are all sensitive to EMFs and limiting and protecting how many you absorb is most likely going to be the subject of many discussions to come in the future, along with products preventing the absorption in our homes and offices and schools. As we get more and more used to the conveniences, it is worth taking a step back and making sure we are not putting our own health in jeopardy for the pleasures of constant Internet access.

Helpful sources on the subject include:

- https://www.healthandenvironment.org
- American Academy of Pediatrics recommendations for children at https://ehtrust.org/american-academy-pediatrics-issues-new -recommendations-reduce-exposure-cell-phones/
- Environmental Health Trust at www.ehtrust.org
- World Health Organization at http://www.who.int/mediacentre /factsheets/fs193/en/
- Healthydwellings.com

CHAPTER 17

HIDDEN TOXINS IN OUR CHILDREN'S TOYS AND CRAFTS

OUR CHILDREN'S toys should be the last thing we worry about. A parent should be able to purchase a toy and not worry about his or her child getting lead poisoning from it. There are regulations, but the issue is that no one is policing them. The goal is to get everything to market as quickly as possible, and what you and I don't know won't hurt us—until it does. My son is ten years old, but I still have to monitor his toys; most recently, his fidget spinner tested positive for lead.

BPAs, mercury, and arsenic, are all found in toys, including the wooden ones that you would not expect. The hardest part of this is there is no obvious source. I went through a *Forbes* article showing the fourteen worst toys as designated by ecocenter.org, which truly surprised me. The article by William Pentland published nine years ago still resonates today.[1]

Here are some of the most surprising findings.

Back when my son was a toddler there were many parents who sub-scribed to the "wooden toy" theory, which was to only give your child nonplastic toys. This seems to be safe, but like anything, it depends on the source. Many wood toys have been treated with chemicals like form-aldehyde or are painted with paints containing leads. The primary colors red and blue, often associated with kids' toys, are also the colors that tend to have the highest lead and cadmium content. Soft, plush stuffed ani-mals are regularly sprayed with flame retardants, which are neurotoxins, and our children sleep with them!

We have to do our own diligence and look at the source and look for brands who advertise what they don't put in.

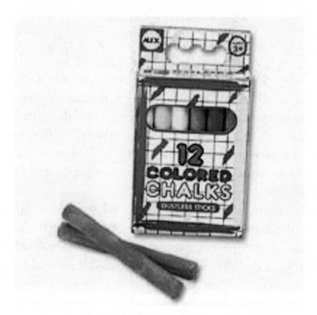

Figure 17.1 12 Colored Chalks, Manufacturer: Alex Panline USA, Inc., Mercury PPM: 423. Source: *Forbes*

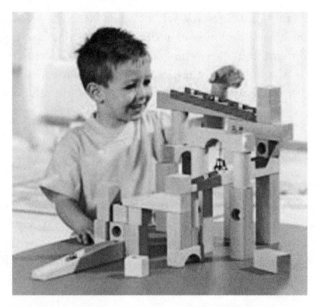

Figure 17.2 Ball Track, Large Basic Set, Manufacturer: Habermaass Corp., Inc., Cadmium PPM: 981
Source: *Forbes*

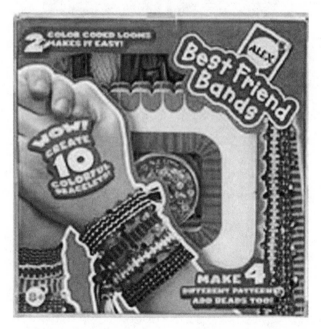

Figure 17.3 Best Friends Band, Manufacturer: Alex Panline USA, Inc., Arsenic PPM: 630
Source: *Forbes*

Here are the guidelines for UL ECOLOGO 172 Certification, as published by UL, a provider of independent testing for manufacturers.[2] Look for toys that carry the ECOLOGO 172 Certification mark, an indication that these toys meet or exceed strict environmental and human health guidelines, helping to ensure toys are safer for children and the environment (see Figure 17.4).

What is ECOLOGO Certification exactly? Here is a description that UL provided for publication.

The UL ECOLOGO 172 standard is a third-party, lifecycle-based, environmental performance standard designed to reduce environmental and human health impacts of toys by specifying criteria for: chemicals, recycled and recyclable materials, sustainably sourced materials, reduced energy use, and minimized pollution

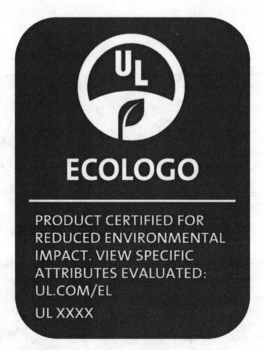

Figure 17.4
Source: UL.COM

generated by the production, use, and disposal of toy products and their packaging. Products that achieve certification to this standard earn the right to carry the UL ECOLOGO certification mark.

Many kids love to do dressup and wear makeup. My son had a brief fascination with nail polish in kindergarten and enjoyed blue toenails. I am glad he grew out of it simply because nail polish is not good for his nails, even those deemed safer for children. There are many makeups and nail polishes saying they are safe to use on little fingers and toes, but I was kind of shocked at what they are calling "natural." One popular brand on the market says their product is: "specially formulated from God's natural ingredients and dries to a hard, durable finish." I was really taken aback at what they call natural. The ingredients in their nail polish are: Water, acrylates copolymer, neem oil. May contain the following colorants (depending on shade): Red 34 Lake, ultramarines, iron oxide, titanium dioxide, mica, red 28, yellow 10, violet 2, zinc sulfide/copper, copper flake, orange 5, and red 22.

The only natural ingredients in this product made by "God" or Mother Nature are Water, Neem Oil, mica, copper flake, zinc sulfide/copper, and iron oxide. The rest are all definitely synthetic and made by humans. As I have mentioned before, natural does not necessarily mean good either, and although there are many colorants that come from the earth, they can still be contaminated with lead, arsenic, and talc. Copper flakes are not something I would want my child eating off of his fingernails either. The main ingredient in this "natural" nail polish is not natural at all. Acrylic copolymer is a chemical binder and is used in nail polishes, hair sprays, and so on to make them stick. Not surprisingly, you can see other products on their site that are also "natural" and indeed are not.

This is a great example of "green washing," and until this gets better policed by the FDA or another organization, we will have to be our own advocates.

This company is far from the only one pushing the boundaries of natural. The cleaning industry of which I am a part and the beauty market all do this. I fully acknowledge that my own products are more than 90 percent derived from natural ingredients, but they are also chemicals. They are safer chemicals because not everything can be made naturally and requires the help of synthetic ingredients. I am not opposed to this; however, cleaning your table and what your child puts on their skin are two very different things. I just don't want you thinking it is "good" for your child.

And what about those special occasions like Halloween?

A few years ago there was lead found in Halloween makeup marketed for kids. This included lip balms, which of course get into their little mouths.[3] The makeup is not required to be tested, and the only reason it was found was because an environmental group in Oregon decided to test it. What about face painting at carnivals and parties? It absolutely has the same potential to have lead and cadmium and other toxins as well.

Removable tattoos are another fun item kids love, but how safe are they? Interestingly I could find little info on them. Just articles saying if they are made in the United States, which means they have to fall under our safety rules using FDA-approved cosmetic colorants. Most are made in China and overseas, which is anyone's guess if they are following U.S. rules.

I did, however, find big warnings for getting henna tattoos or mendhis. These are the intricate designs usually done on hands and are often found in tourist areas. When I went to Morocco, there were several women trying to get my group to get one. Good thing we passed because not all natural henna tattoos use henna. Some use a black hair dye, which causes severe skin reactions, and in some cases, permanent scarring. The ingredient is called PPD and has been banned in skin care ingredients here.[4]

As mentioned in the chapter on clothing, costume jewelry is a huge concern, particularly children's costume jewelry. From charm bracelets, princess crowns, name necklaces, and police badges, these have all been shown to be sources for repeatedly abusing our lead content regulations. Given that young children wear these and often put them in their mouths, I would always do a swab test on any piece of fake jewelry I let my child wear or play with. Of all the concerns mentioned, costume jewelry is truly in need of much higher regulations and enforcement. No amount of lead is safe for their little developing brains.

PLASTIC TOYS

Plastic toys are everywhere in the toy aisles. There is no escaping them. You may not have them at home, but the school or friend's playroom, even the doctor's office will probably have them. The concerns with plastic toys are the exposure to BPAs, phthalates, and lead.

You would have to put your child in a bubble (a nonplastic one at that) to keep them away entirely from plastic. What I recommend is washing their hands after playing with them, which is a good practice to minimize germs and to not let them put them in their mouths. Take a look at Table 17.1 from www.bearsforhumanity.com because it does a good job of listing the concerns and what to ask for when shopping for toys.[5] Toys are a big business and the more we demand it, the more manufacturers will regulate their manufacturing practices and give us what we want.

ART SUPPLIES

Crayons, purple markers that smell like grapes, and glue sticks—who doesn't love a good craft project? There are many safe products out there and the toxic ones like rubber cement are already well known to be toxic and not recommended for kids use. A few shockers, like the purple markers that smell like grapes, can contain xylene, a neuro-, kidney, reproductive, and respiratory toxin.[6] Proper clay that is used in a kiln is made from silica, which when in its loose form is a respiratory concern and a potential carcinogen. Workers in mines wear protective masks, and little children should not be near loose powder. Make sure you also do not inhale the tiny particles. Children should only be given wet clay and be kept away from an active kiln, which can release toxins while the glaze is firing. If they are big playdough lovers—and who isn't—I recommend you make your own or shop one of the natural sources.[7] As it says in SafeMama's blog, there is nothing natural about neon-colored playdough, and we all know so many kids eat it. Best to stay safe and make your own. Lastly glue. We all know you shouldn't sniff rubber cement and that kids often die from huffing it. Rule of

Table 17.1

Uses	Hazardous Chemicals	Possible Health Effects	Used in Products
Various dyes and pigments	Aniline	Very toxic, carcinogenic, and mutagenic	Dolls
Various dyes and pigments	Azocolorants	Carcinogenic, causes allergies	Dolls, cuddly toys, wooden toys, plastic
Dyes and pigments: creates the red, orange, and yellow pigments	Cadmium	Carcinogenic, toxic by inhalation, impairs fertility, disrupts development of children's brains	Dolls, wooden toys, plastic
Dyes and pigments: creates the green, orange, and yellow pigments	Chromium	Carcinogenic, mutagenic, toxic: causes severe burns, impairs fertility	Dolls, cuddly toys, wooden toys, electronic toys
Dyes and pigments: creates the red, orange, and yellow pigments	Lead	Carcinogenic and impairs fertility, effects the developing brain	Dolls, wooden toys, plastic, electronic toys
Fire retardant	Brominated flame retardants	Persistent, bio-accumulative, toxic; some kinds are also classified as carcinogenic, toxic, disrupting the reproductive system; some disrupt the hormone system	Dolls, cuddly toys, plastic, electronic toys
Bind pigments to the cloth; fire retardant; wrinkle resistance; water repellence.; adhesive in wood products	Formaldehydes and formaldehyde releasers (e.g., benzylhemiformal, 2-bromo-2-nitropropane-1,3-diol, 5-bromo-5-nitro-1,3-dioxane, diazolidinyl urea, Imidazolidinyl urea, Quaternium-15, DMDM Hydantoin).	Irritates mucus membranes and skin, can cause hypersensitivity, carcinogenic (nasal pathway)	Cuddly and wooden toys

Uses	Hazardous Chemicals	Possible Health Effects	Used in Products
Water, grease, and soil repellents	Perfluorinated chemicals (PFC)	Carcinogenic, disrupts fertility	Dolls, cuddly toys
A main component in the manufacture of polycarbonate plastics, epoxies, and epoxy resin	Bisphenol-A (BPA)	Disrupts the reproductive and hormone system, increases the risk of cancer	Dolls, plastic, electronic toys
Plastic stabilizer; surfactant in processing textiles	Nonylphenol (ethoxylates)	Endocrine disruptor, persistent— accumulates in the environment	Dolls, cuddly toys, plastic
Plastic stabilizer, usually found in clear plastic	Organotin compounds	Irritates the eyes and skin, toxic to the reproductive system, if ingested is harmful to the central nervous system, endocrine system and reproductive system	Dolls, cuddly toys, wooden toys, plastic
Plasticizer	Chlorinated paraffins	Carcinogenic, disrupts the hormone system	Dolls, plastic, electronic toys
Plasticizer, usually found in soft plastic, pellets for stuffing cuddly toys; can also be used as a synthetic fragrance compound in scented toys	Phthalates	Disrupts development and the hormone system, impairs fertility	Dolls, cuddly toys, plastic and electronic toys
Antibacterial agent	Triclosan	Can cause allergies and bacterial resistance, disrupts the endocrine system	Dolls, cuddly toys, and plastic

thumb: if it smells toxic it is toxic; keep the scented glues away from kids and use white glue or paste.

How do we detox? A child needs toys to develop and learn, and of course, we cannot take them away. Here are a few steps I take to ensure the safety of my son's toys.

1. Buy lead swabs. You can do your own simple lead test at home with handy lead swabs available online. I got them at Amazon.[8] Although it won't tell you how much lead is in the toy, it will tell you if it is present.
2. Always pretest jewelry that is not sterling or gold before gifting it or letting a child wear it, and this includes gold plated or sterling plated. Unless it is marked pure 14k, 18k, 24k, or 925 (which is sterling), always test it. The only exception would be pure stone beads, which to my knowledge have no contamination concerns. And a note on the natural amber necklaces that are being sold as natural teething devices. Please read Jennifer Taylor's informative article because natural or not, they can choke your child.[9]
3. Write the manufacturer. When in doubt, e-mail the manufacturer. All brands have to have a contact and this can usually be found on their website. Ask them if they treat the foam in their stuffed animals with flame retardants. Ask them what their plastics are treated with. I find it shocking that some toys are treated with antibacterial sprays like Triclosan.
4. Buy toys from green toy manufacturers. There are many out there now, and they list all the ingredients they use and what they don't. Check the resources section at the end of this book for some suggestions.
5. Practice hand washing. This has so many benefits! After playing, make it hand-washing time. My son knows that after he plays with a fidget spinner or toys or crafts to wash his hands. This will ensure that when the hands go to the eyes or the mouth (or the nose), that nothing is transferred. This is how most illnesses are transferred by the way, by our hands touching our eyes, nose, or mouth.

CHAPTER 18

MATTRESSES, PILLOWS, AND PAINT

Toxins in Places Where You Would Least Expect It

WHO WOULD have ever thought that our mattresses could be a concern for our thyroids? Or that lead paint is still for sale and readily available? How about that picture frame you just bought, did you stop to wonder whether it had lead in it?

Hidden toxins are everywhere, so much so I couldn't cover them all. Here are a few I uncovered, and I encourage you to be your own sleuth and do your own research. Uncovering and exposing them for all of our health is a job each one of us needs to take on.

LEAD IN YOUR LAWN

Chances are you haven't given your mattress, pillow, or porch a second thought—no more than you have given any thought that your front lawn may have high amounts of lead in the soil. But it probably does. Lead does not biodegrade; once it is there it stays, and most lawns have a moderate amount. This comes from the renovations of older homes with lead paint on the outside—all that dust goes onto lawns and does not wash away with the rain.[1] Cars and their gasoline exhaust are another source of how lead gets into our soil. And if you live next to any sort of manufacturing plant, levels can get so high it is considered hazardous waste.[2]

Before you plant your vegetable garden, it is worth a soil test to make sure your levels are not on the high side. If renovating or buying a new "old" home, have the soil tested. If you find lead, do not live in the home during renovation and make sure the dust is prevented from blowing on to your lawn, your neighbors, and those who live around you.

MATTRESSES AND PILLOWS

So, what about your mattress? Like furniture, they are treated with chemicals to prevent fire. Remember this was a law that was successfully lobbied by the tobacco industry in the 1970s when the government asked them to create a safer cigarette as people were falling asleep with them. Instead they doused our furniture and mattresses with chemicals, including children's cribs. Chemicals that are known carcinogens and mutagens that have affected our health and our planet's health. Billions of pounds of flame-retardant chemicals are manufactured every year. This translates to billions of dollars for an industry that has absolutely no plans to lose that annual income. In fact, they spend millions of dollars creating ad campaigns to convince you the consumer that these chemicals are keeping you safe. They are not. Many of their testimonies in court have be proven to be false statements, including one where a doctor testified a child died from the mother accidentally tipping a candle into the crib and that the lack of flame retardants were the reason the child died. It never happened. This is an industry who silently created and manufactured their own organization—posing as concerned consumers. Firemen have testified that flame retardants don't work, and in fact when they burn, they produce harmful chemicals that make it harder to put out the fire.[3]

California has removed mandatory flame retardants, but they still exist and they are not safer. Chemicals such as Tris, which were banned in the 1970s, are still being used.

All mattresses—except when they advertise otherwise—are treated with fire retardants, even organic ones. The gases released from the chemicals are unseen but real. Your cotton mattress cover is not preventing anything. According to this article from *Healthy Child*, the plastic mattress covers provide some barrier but not enough.[4] Considering we spend 30 percent of our life in bed, we absolutely should make sure our mattresses are not leaching chemicals. In fact, we should demand it. If you do anything, make sure your children's mattresses are free of flame retardants. Also check their changing pads, blankets, and strollers. Cotton and wool are all good options and the *Healthy Child* article provides many good resources that are the same cost as a regular, chemically treated mattress. There are also wonderful, family owned sources found at the end of this book. I recommend you watch the informational videos created by Arlene Blum, a chemist and the woman we can thank for exposing the truth about harmful flame-retardant chemicals back in the mid-1970s, at http://www.sixclasses.org/. Blum has tirelessly worked to get the chemicals banned and off our furniture for more than four decades now.

Pillows made of foam or polyfill are also subject to regulations. Polyfill is flammable and is usually treated when used in pillows and blankets. Opt for an organic wool or cotton pillow.[5]

Real down makes for an excellent pillow, but the way the feathers are resourced will make your skin crawl. Down is often gathered off of live birds where the feathers are plucked and pulled off of a screaming duck. It is one of the most disturbing processes I have personally seen. When it comes to coats, the other option is polyfill, which could be treated with flame retardants. It is all enough to make you move to a hot climate where coats and blankets are not needed. There are companies like Patagonia and North Face who independently audit their sources to make sure the down is gathered humanely. When shopping for bedding, pillows, and clothing look for the responsible down standard (RDS) seal, ensuring that the down is certified ethically sourced.

When shopping for any bedding, make sure it is free of flame retardants. There are some organic products that are still doused with it. Always ask!

PAINT

Like flame-retardant chemicals that were banned then allowed again, so is lead paint. Lead paint was banned in the United States in 1977—but only in consumer paints. Lead paint is still used in some commercial paints like the white lines on roads, the metal on buildings, and more.[6]

In other countries, it is much worse, according to this 2014 study, consumer paints in Africa are filled with lead paint still, as are many other countries including India, China, Mexico, and Argentina.[7]

If you purchase products from these countries, you should expect the paint to have lead in it. For the United States a Q&A from the EPA, which tells you how lead is regulated and what your rights are, is a good source.[8] Also note that most children are exposed to lead via dust—not eating paint chips. So the concern should definitely not dissipate once your child has passed the toddler stage. If you have lead paint in your home, every time you clean it, you are exposing yourself and your family to the dust and potential lead poisoning.

GARDEN HOSES

Having spent years of my life drinking from a garden hose and running around in a sprinkler like so many suburban kids today, I was so sad to find this information. Garden hoses are a big source of phthalates and the heat of the sun on the hose makes them a toxic water faucet for your kids. A 2016 "Garden Hose Study" by ecocenter.org is comprehensive enough for me to look for a safer hose for my kids, my pets, and my garden, which is watered with a hose.[9] All of the hoses were purchased at stores you and I shop in and are regularly available online. Even some of the metal tops had lead in them, which is exactly where a person puts their mouths to take a sip. Of all the hoses tested, the ones that had the least concerns were the non-PVC hoses. They may be less flexible, but sometimes we need to trade off convenience for our better health.

IN SUMMARY

THIS BOOK has been an honor and a gift to write. We are living in a world where many of our leaders and elected officials are sacrificing their own morals and, dare I say, souls for personal power and gain. I am grateful for my own awakening to the toxins in this world and the determination to make our world a healthier place for us all to live in.

There are many times in writing this book I screamed, I cried, and I posted on Facebook the horrific findings I came across. It is hard to believe that any person in their right mind would allow a toxin to be used and sold to the public. I simply cannot understand how anyone can tell themselves it is okay, when they know fully well that it is harming and potentially killing another human. But I should not be shocked because for years I was a smoker without concern. It is a decision I profoundly regret, but it is also a lesson to the power of our minds. We can convince ourselves of anything—for better or for worse.

The information I found and received while writing this book was hard to bear, but it also gave me power and clarity. As I write, the U.S. president is in the process of dismantling the EPA and deregulating our clean water act. He is opening up the floodgates for more and more toxins to come in and removing the repercussions to the corporations who dump it. Every day is a new nightmare. But I feel more hopeful than ever because I know the power to solve this is not—and never was—with our elected officials. The power is with you and me. But there is one caveat; we must speak out. You cannot expect a knight-in-shining-armor to rescue our planet; it is not going to happen. But you can open your laptop and write an e-mail to make a difference. There are many amazing organizations and people doing good work—decades of good work—and they would love for you to join them. Encourage your children and grandchildren to grow up and create technology that will bring us innovation, jobs, and sustainability—like solar power—which is now cheaper than electricity.

I have a huge amount of hope for my son and his generation. They will have a lot to fix, but they will not be without work. They will create the new world we seek, because they will have no choice. The writing is already on the wall, one in two of us will get cancer. The ramifications of industrialization and the lack of regulations for more than half a century are here. We see it in our own health, with nearly every person I know suffering from an autoimmune disease.

There are many who will resist it, but once they see better jobs and a healthier life, they will gladly join. I am delighted and in awe to know persons like Jonathan Webb, who took it upon himself to create a new economy for his fellow Appalachians with the creation of Appharvest.co. Providing local and nutritious foods, jobs, and a new life to a state that has been economically depressed for years. And not just a job, but good jobs, where they will work in healthy conditions for themselves, creating healthy foods for their families. This idea came from one person with gumption and a heart to do the right thing.

This is the future, this is the new paradigm.

We are all a part of this, and it is through the efforts of each one of us, we will make a difference. A phone call, a decision to not buy bottled water, or the creation of a truly humane and sustainable company all are needed.

It is an honor to witness and be a part of this movement for health and I thank you for your part in being the change we seek.

Be well.

RESOURCES

HAIR CARE, FACE CREAMS, MAKEUP, AND DENTAL PRODUCTS

www.100percentpure.com
www.tammyfender.com
www.oseamalibu.com
www.credobeauty.com
www.davids-usa.com
www.schmidtsdeodorant.com
www.juicebeauty.com
www.gemstoneorganic.com
https://madebyradius.com
www.jason-personalcare.com
https://yarokhair.com

HOUSEHOLD PRODUCTS

www.bambuhome.com
www.skoy.com
www.lodge.com
www.northerngrade.com
www.rodales.com
http://www.emersoncreekpottery.com
http://www.hfcoors.com
https://www.fiestafactorydirect.com
www.mountainvalleyspring.com

CLOTHING AND ACCESSORIES

https://www.nortonpoint.com (Sunglasses)
www.hardtailforever.com (Made in the United States workout wear)
www.patagonia.com (Clothing and outer wear)
http://featheredfriends.com (RDS down outerwear)
https://wearpact.com (Underwear and socks)
http://study-ny.com (Clothing)
http://www.jsbrooklyn.com (Handmade and affordable sandals)
https://www.simulacra.nyc (Clothing)
https://www.tm1985.com (Beautiful leather travel bags)
http://www.bluerdenim.com (Jeans)
http://www.greeneileen.org (Repurposed/resale clothing)
https://www.thereformation.com (Clothing)
https://www.indigenous.com (Organic and indigenous wool sweaters)
http://nuiorganics.com (Kids clothing)
www.wearethought.com (Clothing)
https://zshoesorganic.com (Shoes)
https://www.allbirds.com (Shoes)
https://www.solerebels.com (Shoes)

MATTRESSES AND PILLOWS

http://dashingstarfarm.com (Chemical free, wool bedding and pillows, small and privately owned)
http://www.surroundewe.com (Organic wool mattresses and bedding small and privately owned)
http://featheredfriends.com (RDS down bedding)
https://www.downlinens.com (RDS-certified down bedding)
https://www.thecleanbedroom.com (Organic cotton, latex, and wool mattresses)

TOYS

https://bannortoys.com
https://elvesandangels.com
https://smilingtreetoys.com/

https://unclegoose.com
https://www.palumba.com

SUGGESTED READING

A World without Cancer by Margaret I. Cuomo, MD; also a PBS special
    of the same name
We the Eaters by Ellen Gustafson
When Corporations Rule the World by David C. Korten
Farmacology by Dr. Daphne Miller
Bringing It to the Table" by Wendell Berry
What Causes Cancer? What We Know and What It Means by Anthony B.
    Miller, MD, FRCP, FRCP(C), FHPHM, FACE

SUGGESTED SITES

http://greensciencepolicy.org/
www.safecosmetics.org
https://www.healthandenvironment.org
https://www.ncbi.nlm.nih.gov
http://www.ngocsd-ny.org
http://sierraclub.org/

NOTES

LABELS AND REGULATORS

1. Ronald E. Gordon, Sean Fitzgerald, and James Millette, "Asbestos in commercial cosmetic talcum powder as a cause of mesothelioma in women." *International Journal of Occupational and Environmental Health* 20(4), (2014 Oct): 318–32, doi: 10.1179/2049396714Y.0000000081

2. "High-Risk Crops & Inputs." Non-GMO Project Standard website. Accessed July 19, 2017, from https://www.nongmoproject.org/gmo-facts/high-risk/.

3. Different action thresholds exist for compliant seed used to grow livestock feed. See Table 4 in Section VII.A.2 of "Non-GMO Project Standard: Version 14.1." Non-GMO Project website, May 19, 2017. Accessed July 18, 2017, from https://www.nongmoproject.org/wp-content/uploads/2017/07/Non-GMO-Project-Standard-Version-14.1_5-18-17.pdf.

PART I

DETOX YOUR SKIN

1. Gina McCarthy, "TSCA Reform: A Bipartisan Milestone to Protect Our Health from Dangerous Chemicals" *The EPA Blog*, June 22, 2016, https://blog.epa.gov/blog/2016/06/tsca-reform-a-bipartisan-milestone-to-protect-our-health-from-dangerous-chemicals/.

CHAPTER 1

1. C. Liao, F. Liu, and K. Kannan, "Occurrence of and dietary exposure to parabens in foodstuffs from the United States." *Environmental Science & Technology*, 47(8), (2013 Apr 16): 3918–25, doi: 10.1021/es400724s.

2. "Propyl Paraben in Drinking Water." Environmental Health Division, Minnesota Department of Health. Accessed July 13, 2017, from http://www .health.state.mn.us/divs/eh/risk/guidance/dwec/propylparainfo.pdf.

3. C. L. Burnett, et al., "Final report of the safety assessment of methylisothiazolinone." *International Journal of Toxicology*, 29(4 Suppl) (2010 Jul): 187S–213S, doi: 10.1177/1091581810374651.

4. Rachel Abrams, "Growing Scrutiny for an Allergy Trigger Used in Personal Care Products." *New York Times*, January 23, 2015. Accessed July 13, 2017, from https://www.nytimes.com/2015/01/24/business/allergy-trigger-found-in -many-personal-care-items-comes-under-greater-scrutiny.html.

5. "Cancer chemical found in drinks." *BBC News*, Last Updated: Wednesday, 1 March 2006, 18:38 GMT. Accessed July 13, 2017, from http://news .bbc.co.uk/2/hi/health/4763528.stm.

6. ToxServices Toxicology Risk Assessment Consulting, "GreenScreen(tm) Assessment for Sodium Benzoate (CAS #532-32-1)." Report prepared for Clean Production Action, Washington, D.C., December 11, 2012, http:// www.healthandenvironment.org/docs/532-32-1_Sodium_benzoate_GS-100_ v1.2_Dec_2012.pdf.

7. European Chemicals Agency, "Proposal for Harmonised Classification and Labelling: Potassium Sorbate (CAS Number: 24634-61-5)." Report submitted by Germany, November 2011, https://echa.europa.eu/ documents/10162/13626/clh_potassium_sorbate_en.pdf.

8. Shanna H. Swan, "Environmental phthalate exposure in relation to reproductive outcomes and other health endpoints in humans." *Environmental Research*, 108(2), (2008 Oct): 177–84, doi: 10.1016/j.envres.2008.08.007.

9. Rishikesh Mankidy, et al., "Biological impact of phthalates." *Toxicology Letters*, 217, (2013): 50–58, http://www.usask.ca/toxicology/jgiesy/pdf/ publications/JA-712.pdf.

CHAPTER 2

1. Say No to Palm Oil website, http://www.saynotopalmoil.com, accessed July 13, 2017.

2. M. St. J. Warne, and A. D. Schifko, "Toxicity of laundry detergent components to a freshwater cladoceran and their contribution to detergent toxicity." *Ecotoxicology and Environmental Safety*, 44(2), (1999 Oct): 196–206, doi: 10.1006/eesa.1999.1824.

3. California Safe Cosmetics Program, "Reportable Ingredients List." *Sacramento: California Department of Public Health—Occupational Health Branch*, 2016. Accessed July 13, 2017, from https://archive.cdph.ca.gov/programs /cosmetics/Documents/chemlist.pdf.

4. Alison Kodjak, "FDA Bans 19 Chemicals Used in Antibacterial Soaps." *Shots: Health News From NPR*, September 2, 201612:56 PM ET. Accessed July 13, 2017, from http://www.npr.org/sections/health-shots/2016/09/02 /492394717/fda-bans-19-chemicals-used-in-antibacterial-soaps.

5. Megan Gannon, "Triclosan, found in antibacterial soap and other products, causes cancer in mice." *Washington Post*, November 24, 2014. Accessed July 13, 2017, from https://www.washingtonpost.com/national/health-science /triclosan-found-in-antibacterial-soap-and-other-products-causes-cancer-in-mice /2014/11/24/096b8ca4-70cc-11e4-ad12-3734c461eab6_story.html?utm _term=.f6da1f63a6ae.

6. Annmarie Skin Care, "Ingredient Watch List: Cyclotetrasiloxane, the Hair Conditioner That May Harm Our Waterways." Accessed July 13, 2017, from https://www.annmariegianni.com/ingredient-watch-list-cyclotetrasiloxane-the -hair-conditioner-that-may-harm-our-waterways/.

7. Andalou Naturals website. Accessed July 13, 2017, from www.andalou .com.

8. Avalon Organics website. Accessed July 13, 2017, from www.avalon organics.com.

9. Juice Organics website. Accessed July 13, 2017, from www.juiceorganics .com.

CHAPTER 3

1. "FDA's Testing of Cosmetics for Arsenic, Cadmium, Chromium, Cobalt, Lead, Mercury, and Nickel Content." *U.S. Food & Drug Administration*, updated: 12/21/2016. Accessed July 13, 2017, from https://www.fda.gov/ Cosmetics/ProductsIngredients/PotentialContaminants/ucm452836.htm.

2. "Toxicology and Carcinogenesis Studies of Talc (CAS No. 14807-96-6) (Non-Asbestiform) in F344/N Rats and B6C3F1 Mice (Inhalation Studies)." Research Triangle Park, NC: National Toxicology Program, September 1993. Accessed July 13, 2017, from https://ntp.niehs.nih.gov/ntp/htdocs/lt_rpts/ tr421.pdf.

3. Associated Press, "Johnson & Johnson to pay $72m in case linking baby powder to ovarian cancer." *The Guardian*, February 23, 2016. Accessed July 13, 2017, from https://www.theguardian.com/world/2016/feb/24/ johnson-johnson-72-millon-babuy-talcum-powder-ovarian-cancer.

4. P. A. Leggat and U. Kedjarune, "Toxicity of Methyl Methacrylate in Dentistry." *International Dental Journal*, 53(3), (June 2003): 126–31, PMID: 12873108.

5. "FD&C Blue No.1." *Food Additives World*. Accessed July 13, 2017, from http://www.foodadditivesworld.com/fdc-blue-no1.html.

6. Keely Chalmers, "Tests find toxic metals in children's Halloween makeup." *USA Today Network* (Portland, Oregon: KGW-TV, October 26, 2016). Accessed July 19, 2017, from https://www.usatoday.com/story /news/nation-now/2016/10/26/toxic-metals-childrens-halloween-makeup /92759186/.

7. Adriana Dehelean and Dana Alina Magdas, "Analysis of Mineral and Heavy Metal Content of Some Commercial Fruit Juices by Inductively Coupled Plasma Mass Spectrometry." *Scientific World Journal* (December 2013), doi: 10.1155/2013/215423.

8. Ibrahim M. Aldjain, et al., "Determination of Heavy Metals in the Fruit of Date Palm Growing at Different Locations of Riyadh." *Saudi Journal of Biological Sciences*, 18(2), (2011): 175–80, doi: 10.1016/j.sjbs.2010.12.001.

9. Gina L. LoSasso, et al., "Neurocognitive Sequelae of Exposure to Organic Solvents and (Meth)Acrylates among Nail-Studio Technicians." *Cognitive and Behavioral Neurology*, 15(1), (March 2002): 44–55. Accessed July 13, 2017, from http://journals.lww.com/cogbehavneurol/pages/articleviewer.aspx ?year=2002&issue=03000&article=00007&type=abstract.

CHAPTER 4

1. Global Industry Analysts, Inc., "Global Toothpaste Market to Reach US$12.6 Billion by 2015, According to New Report by Global Industry Analysts, Inc." *PRWeb*, October 19, 2010. Accessed July 13, 2017, from http://www.prweb.com/releases/toothpaste_oral_care/whitening_regular /prweb4661914.htm.

2. R. S. Lanigan, "Final Report on the Safety Assessment of Sodium Metaphosphate, Sodium Trimetaphosphate, and Sodium Hexametaphosphate." *International Journal of Toxicology*, 20 Suppl 3 (2001): 75–89, PMID: 11766135.

3. Joanne K. Tobacman, "Review of Harmful Gastrointestinal Effects of Carrageenan in Animal Experiments." *Environmental Health Perspectives*, 109(10), (2001): 983–94. Accessed July 13, 2017, from https://www.ncbi.nlm .nih.gov/pmc/articles/PMC1242073/pdf/ehp0109-000983.pdf.

4. Paul Connett, "50 Reasons to Oppose Fluoridation." *FluorideAlert.org*, updated September 2012. Accessed July 13, 2017, from http://fluoridealert.org/ articles/50-reasons/.

5. Douglas Main, "Fluoridation May Not Prevent Cavities, Scientific Review Shows." *Newsweek*, June 29, 2015. Accessed July 13, 2017, from http:// www.newsweek.com/fluoridation-may-not-prevent-cavities-huge-study-shows -348251.

6. "Xylitol: Should We Stop Calling It Natural?" *Crunchy Betty*, last updated on June 19, 2017. Accessed July 13, 2017, from https://crunchybetty. com/xylitol-should-we-stop-calling-it-natural/.

7. Alison Kodjak, "FDA Bans 19 Chemicals Used in Antibacterial Soaps." *Shots: Health News From NPR*, September 2, 2016 12:56 PM ET. Accessed July 13, 2017, from http://www.npr.org/sections/health-shots/2016/09/02/492394717/fda-bans-19-chemicals-used-in-antibacterial-soaps.

8. J. A. Camargo, "Fluoride Toxicity to Aquatic Organisms: A review." *Chemosphere*, 50(3), (2003): 251–64, PMID: 12656244.

9. "Colgate Total® Toothpaste and the Environment." *Colgate-Palmolive Company*. Accessed July 13, 2017, from http://www.colgatetotal.com/health-benefits/colgate-total-toothpaste-and-the-environment.

10. A. Albert-Kiszely, et al., "Comparison of the effects of cetylpyridinium chloride with an essential oil mouth rinse on dental plaque and gingivitis—a six-month randomized controlled clinical trial." *Journal of Clinical Periodontology*, 34(8), (2007): 658–68, doi: 10.1111/j.1600-051X.2007.01103.x.

11. "Potassium pyrophosphate." *PubChem Open Chemistry Database*, PubChem CID: 23740, create date: August 8, 2005. Accessed July 13, 2017, from https://pubchem.ncbi.nlm.nih.gov/compound/Potassium_pyrophosphate #section=Health-Hazard.

12. "How to Whiten Teeth Naturally with Turmeric." *Mommypotamus*. Accessed July 13, 2017, from https://www.mommypotamus.com/whiten-teeth -naturally-turmeric/.

13. "The Pros and Cons of Floss Choices." *Oral-B*. Accessed July 19, 2017, from https://oralb.com/en-us/oral-care-topics/the-pros-and-cons-of-floss-choices.

14. The American Cancer Society medical and editorial content team, "Teflon and Perfluorooctanoic Acid (PFOA)." *American Cancer Society*, last revised: January 5, 2016. Accessed July 13, 2017, from https://www.cancer.org/cancer/cancer-causes/teflon-and-perfluorooctanoic-acid-pfoa.html.

CHAPTER 5

1. "Frequently asked questions on genetically modified foods." *World Health Organization*, published May 2014. Accessed July 19, 2017, from http://www.who.int/foodsafety/areas_work/food-technology/faq-genetically -modified-food/en/.

2. Shireen Karimi, "Another Strike Against GMOs—The Creation of Superbugs and Superweeds." *GMOInside.org*. Accessed July 13, 2017, from http://www.gmoinside.org/another-strike-gmos-creation-superbugs-superweeds/.

3. Theresa Papademetriou, "Restrictions on Genetically Modified Organisms: European Union." *The Law Library of Congress*, last updated June 9, 2015. Accessed July 13, 2017, from http://www.loc.gov/law/help/restrictions-on-gmos/eu.php.

4. Marian Burros, "Study Finds Far Less Pesticide Residue on Organic Produce." *The New York Times*, May 8, 2002. Accessed July 13, 2017, from http://

www.nytimes.com/2002/05/08/us/study-finds-far-less-pesticide-residue-on
-organic-produce.html.

5. Tamar Haspel, "Is organic better for your health? A look at milk, meat, eggs, produce and fish," *The Washington Post*, April 7, 2014. Accessed July 13, 2017, from https://www.washingtonpost.com/national/health-science/is
-organic-better-for-your-health-a-look-at-milk-meat-eggs-produce-and-fish/
2014/04/07/036c654e-a313-11e3-8466-d34c451760b9_story.html?tid=a_
inl&utm_term=.eb571a1afd7d.

6. "Demeter International." *Wikipedia, The Free Encyclopedia*. Accessed July 13, 2017, from https://en.wikipedia.org/w/index.php?title=Demeter
_International&oldid=780919492.

7. "Biodynamic agriculture." *Wikipedia, The Free Encyclopedia*. Accessed July 13, 2017, from https://en.wikipedia.org/w/index.php?title=Biodynamic_
agriculture&oldid=788736112.

CHAPTER 6

1. Julie M. Rodriguez, "44% of US honeybee colonies died off last year." *Inhabitat*, May 13, 2016. Accessed July 13, 2017, from http://inhabitat.com/
honeybees-are-still-dying-off-at-record-rates/.

2. Miguel A. Altieri, et al., "Crops, weeds and pollinators: Understanding ecological interaction for better management." *Food and Agriculture Organization of the United Nations*, Rome 2015: 2. Accessed July 19, 2017, from http://
www.fao.org/3/a-i3821e.pdf.

3. "List of crop plants pollinated by bees." Available at https://en.wiki-pedia.org/w/index.php?title=List_of_crop_plants_pollinated_by_bees&oldid
=789966192.

4. "EPA Actions to Protect Pollinators." *U.S. Environmental Protection Agency*. Accessed July 13, 2017, from https://www.epa.gov/pollinator-protection/
epa-actions-protect-pollinators.

5. "Existing Scientific Evidence of the Effects of Neonicotinoid Pesticides on Bees." *European Parliament Directorate-General for Internal Policies*, Luxembourg: 2012, Catalogue BA-02-13-260-EN-C. Accessed July 19, 2017, from http://www.europarl.europa.eu/RegData/etudes/note/join/2012/492465/
IPOL-ENVI_NT(2012)492465_EN.pdf.

CHAPTER 7

1. Paul Stamets, "Maitake: The Magnificent 'Dancing' Mushroom." *The Huffington Post*, updated May 21, 2013. Accessed July 13, 2017, from http://
www.huffingtonpost.com/paul-stamets/maitake-mushroom_b_2908332.html.

2. Carol Potera, "Diet and Nutrition: The Artificial Food Dye Blues."

Environmental Health Perspectives, 118(10), (2010): A428, doi: 10.1289/ehp.118-a428.

3. "Milk for Your Bones?" *WebMD*, October 6, 2000. Accessed July 13, 2017, from http://www.webmd.com/diet/healthy-kitchen-11/dairy-truths?page=2.

4. Kelsey Gee, "America's Dairy Farmers Dump 43 Million Gallons of Excess Milk." *The Wall Street Journal*, updated Oct. 12, 2016. Accessed July 13, 2017, from https://www.wsj.com/articles/americas-dairy-farmers-dump-43-million-gallons-of-excess-milk-1476284353.

CHAPTER 8

1. Ron Fleming and Marcy Ford, "Human versus Animals—Comparison of Waste Properties." (Research Paper, Ridgetown College, University of Guelph, July 4, 2001.) Accessed July 13, 2017, from http://www.ridgetownc.uoguelph.ca/research/documents/fleming_huvsanim0107.PDF.

2. "What is the biggest source of pollution in the ocean?" *National Ocean Service, National Oceanic and Atmospheric Administration*, U.S. Department of Commerce, revised July 6, 2017. Accessed July 13, 2017, from https://oceanservice.noaa.gov/facts/pollution.html.

3. Laura Parker, "Slimy Green Beaches May Be Florida's New Normal" *National Geographic*, July 27, 2016. Accessed July 13, 2017, from http://news.nationalgeographic.com/2016/07/toxic-algae-florida-beaches-climate-swamp-environment/.

4. "Antibiotic Debate Overview." *Frontline*. Accessed July 13, 2017, from http://www.pbs.org/wgbh/pages/frontline/shows/meat/safe/overview.html.

5. "Factory Farming." *Farm Sanctuary*. Accessed July 13, 2017, from https://www.farmsanctuary.org/learn/factory-farming/.

6. "Becoming a vegetarian." *Harvard Health Publications*, updated March 18, 2016. Accessed July 13, 2017, from http://www.health.harvard.edu/staying-healthy/becoming-a-vegetarian.

7. Jennifer Chait, "Is Organic Livestock Production More Humane Than Conventional?" *The Balance*, updated September 19, 2016. Accessed July 13, 2017, from https://www.thebalance.com/is-organic-livestock-production-more-humane-2538119.

8. "Factory Farming." *Farm Sanctuary*. Accessed July 13, 2017, from https://www.farmsanctuary.org/learn/factory-farming/.

9. Michael Ruhlman, "Why It's Ethical to Eat Meat." *Ruhlman: Translating the Chef's Craft for Every Kitchen*, May 29, 2012. Accessed July 13, 2017, from http://ruhlman.com/2012/05/why-its-ethical-to-eat-meat/.

10. Nick Tabor and James Walsh, "The Omnivore's Guilt Trip." *New York Magazine*, July 11, 2016.

11. "Overfishing." *World Wildlife Fund.* Accessed July 13, 2017, from https://www.worldwildlife.org/threats/overfishing.

12. Celine Serrat, "Taking the environmental bite out of salmon farming." Phys.org, September 28, 2016. Accessed July 13, 2017, from https://phys.org/news/2016-09-environmental-salmon-farming.html.

13. "Vaccinating salmon: How Norway avoids antibiotics in fish farming." *World Health Organization*, October 2015. Accessed July 13, 2017, from http://www.who.int/features/2015/antibiotics-norway/en/.

14. Andrew Pollack, "Genetically Engineered Salmon Approved for Consumption." *The New York Times*, November 19, 2015. Accessed July 13, 2017, from https://www.nytimes.com/2015/11/20/business/genetically-engineered-salmon-approved-for-consumption.html?_r=0.

15. Roddy Scheer and Doug Moss, "How Does Mercury Get into Fish?" *Scientific American*. Accessed July 13, 2017, from https://www.scientificamerican.com/article/how-does-mercury-get-into/.

16. Paul Greenberg, "The Fish on My Plate." *Frontline*, April 25, 2017. Accessed July 13, 2017, from http://www.pbs.org/wgbh/frontline/film/the-fish-on-my-plate/.

17. Ian Urbina, "'Sea Slaves': The Human Misery That Feeds Pets and Livestock." *The New York Times*, July 27, 2015. Accessed July 13, 2017, from https://www.nytimes.com/2015/07/27/world/outlaw-ocean-thailand-fishing-sea-slaves-pets.html.

18. Jessica Boddy, "Are We Eating Our Fleece Jackets? Microfibers Are Migrating into Field and Food." *The Salt: What's on Your Plate,* February 6, 2017. Accessed July 13, 2017, from http://www.npr.org/sections/thesalt/2017/02/06/511843443/are-we-eating-our-fleece-jackets-microfibers-are-migrating-into-field-and-food.

19. Mary Catherine O'Connor, "California's Fish Are Ingesting Tiny Fibers from Your Favorite Jacket." *Outside*, November 3, 2015. Accessed July 13, 2017, from https://www.outsideonline.com/2032231/californias-fish-are-ingesting-tiny-fibers-your-favorite-jacket.

20. "Microbead." *Wikipedia, The Free Encyclopedia.* Accessed July 13, 2017, fromhttps://en.wikipedia.org/w/index.php?title=Microbead&oldid=790483847.

CHAPTER 9

1. Todd C. Frankel, "New NASA data show how the world is running out of water." *The Washington Post*, June 16, 2015. Accessed July 13, 2017, from https://www.washingtonpost.com/news/wonk/wp/2015/06/16/new-nasa-studies-show-how-the-world-is-running-out-of-water/?utm_term=.340c8ccd8364.

2. "Thirsty Food: Fueling Agriculture to Fuel Humans." *National Geographic Environment.* Accessed July 14, 2017, from http://environment.nationalgeographic.com/environment/freshwater/food/.

3. "National Primary Drinking Water Regulations." *U.S. Environmental Protection Agency*, last updated July 11, 2017. Accessed July 14, 2017, from https://www.epa.gov/ground-water-and-drinking-water/national-primary-drinking-water-regulations.

4. WTOL Staff, "'Do not drink, do not boil' water: Crisis closes out second day with little information." WTOL-11 Toledo website, August 2, 2014. Accessed July 14, 2017, from http://www.wtol.com/story/26178506/do-not-drink-do-not-boil-water-advisory-issued-for-issued-for-lucas-county-surrounding-area.

5. Ben Panko, "Scientists Now Know Exactly How Lead Got into Flint's Water." Smithsonian.com, February 3, 2017. Accessed July 14, 2017, from http://www.smithsonianmag.com/science-nature/chemical-study-ground-zero-house-flint-water-crisis-180962030/.

6. Arthur Delaney, "Lots of Cities Have the Same Lead Pipes that Poisoned Flint." *The Huffington Post*, updated February 22, 2016. Accessed July 14, 2017, from http://www.huffingtonpost.com/entry/lead-pipes-everywhere_us_56a8e916e4b0f71799288f54.

7. "Drugs in the water," *Harvard Health Publications*, published June 2011. Accessed July 14, 2017, from http://www.health.harvard.edu/newsletter_article/drugs-in-the-water.

8. Corinne S. Kennedy and Ian James, "Nestle pipes water from national forest, sparking protests." *USAToday Network: The* (Palm Springs, CA) *Desert Sun*, updated April 3, 2017. Accessed July 14, 2017, from https://www.usatoday.com/story/money/nation-now/2017/04/03/nestle-pumps-water-national-forrest-without-paying-sparking-protest/99982518/.

9. *Bottled Life.* Directed by Urs Schnell. Switzerland: DokLab, Eikon-Südwest, et al., 2012.

10. "List of Nestlé Brands." *Wikipedia, The Free Encyclopedia.* Accessed July 14, 2017, from https://en.wikipedia.org/w/index.php?title=List_of_Nestl%C3%A9_brands&oldid=789116202.

11. Julia Lurie, "Bottled Water Comes From the Most Drought-Ridden Places in the Country." *Mother Jones*, Aug. 11, 2014. Accessed July 14, 2017, from http://www.motherjones.com/environment/2014/08/bottled-water-california-drought/.

12. "Phthalates: The Everywhere Chemical." *Zero Breast Cancer* (formerly Marin Breast Cancer Watch), San Rafael, California. Accessed July 14, 2017, from https://www.niehs.nih.gov/research/supported/assets/docs/j_q/phthalates_the_everywhere_chemical_handout_508.pdf.

13. Marianne Marchese, "The Truth about Plastic Water Bottles." *Smart Publications*. Accessed July 14, 2017, from http://www.smart-publications.com/articles/the-truth-about-plastic-water-bottles.

14. Tom Philpott, "The Dangerous Chemical Lurking in Your Beer Can." *Mother Jones*, February 9, 2015. Accessed July 14, 2017, from http://www.motherjones.com/food/2015/02/no-i-cant-why-im-turning-away-canned-craft-beer/.

15. Erin Brockovich, "Protection or Poison? Chloramination of Drinking Water." Vermonters for a Clean Environment website, October 2010. Accessed July 14, 2017, from http://www.vce.org/ErinBrockovichChloramination.html.

CHAPTER 10

1. Kristin L. Kamerud, Kevin A. Hobbie, and Kim A. Anderson, "Stainless Steel Leaches Nickel and Chromium into Foods During Cooking." *Journal of Agricultural and Food Chemistry*, 61(39), (2013): 9495–501, doi: 10.1021/jf402400v.

2. Debra Lynn Dadd, "Stainless Steel Leaching into Food and Beverages." *Live Toxic Free*, January 17, 2010. Accessed July 14, 2017, from http://www.debralynndadd.com/q-a/stainless-steel-leaching-into-food-and-beverages/.

3. "Testing my stuff for lead." *Natural Baby Mamma*, October 27, 2014. Accessed July 14, 2017, from https://thenaturalbabymama.com/toxins/testing-my-stuff-for-lead/.

4. Mariah Blake, "The Scary New Evidence on BPA-Free Plastics." *Mother Jones*, March/April 2014. Accessed July 14, 2017, from http://www.motherjones.com/environment/2014/03/tritan-certichem-eastman-bpa-free-plastic-safe/.

5. Darby Minow Smith, "Composting 101 for City Dwellers." *Grist*, August 13, 2010. Accessed July 14, 2017, from http://grist.org/article/food-composting-101-slideshow/.

CHAPTER 11

1. "The Human Foot Print—Journey of a Life Time." *Green Contributor*. Accessed July 14, 2017, from http://www.greencontributor.com/index.php/human-foot-print.html.

2. Ellen Byron, "The Great American Soap Overdose." *The Wall Street Journal*, updated January 25, 2010. Accessed July 14, 2017, from https://www.wsj.com/articles/SB10001424052748703808904575025021214910714.

3. "Green Laundry Statistics." *Grand Valley State University Student Housing*, last modified March 21, 2014. Accessed July 14, 2017, from https://www.gvsu.edu/housing/students/green-laundry-statistics-59.htm.

4. Emily Main, "Tide Now 'Free & Clear' of Cancer-Causers." *Rodale's Organic Life*, January 29, 2013. Accessed July 14, 2017, from https://www .rodalesorganiclife.com/wellbeing/free-and-clear-detergent.

5. Ibid.

6. "What happens when detergents get into freshwater ecosystems?" *Lenntech BV*. Accessed July 14, 2017, from http://www.lenntech.com/aquatic/ detergents.htm#ixzz3yl693HD7.

7. Ibid.

8. "The Truth about Sulfates." *Best Health Magazine*, November/December 2010. Accessed July 14, 2017, from http://www.besthealthmag.ca/best-looks/ skin/the-truth-about-sulfates/#sIHv88vBuRLlMTQq.99.

9. "Quaternary ammonium cation." *Wikipedia, The Free Encyclopedia*. Accessed July 14, 2017, from https://en.wikipedia.org/w/index.php?title =Quaternary_ammonium_cation&oldid=775121471.

10. "Social and Environmental Impact of Palm Oil." *Wikipedia, The Free Encyclopedia*. Accessed July 14, 2017, from https://en.wikipedia.org/w/index.php ?title=Social_and_environmental_impact_of_palm_oil&oldid=788542658.

11. Karen Peltier, "Why Optical Brightening Chemicals Are Not Needed in Laundry Detergents." *The Spruce*, updated December 26, 2016. Accessed July 14, 2017, from https://www.thespruce.com/optical-brighteners-chemicals -not-needed-1707025.

CHAPTER 12

1. VOCs are organic chemicals that have a high vapor pressure at ordinary room temperature. Their high vapor pressure results from a low boiling point, which causes large numbers of molecules to evaporate or sublimate from the liquid or solid form of the compound and enter the surrounding air. Paint, bleach, and many household products have high VOCs.

2. The study was led by Lidia Casas of the Center for Environment and Health at KU Leuven in Leuven, the Netherlands.

3. "DIETHYLENE TRIAMINE PENTA ACETIC ACID (DTPA)." *MSDS Lab Report*, Mumbai, India: Nile Chemicals. Accessed July 14, 2017, from http://www.nilechemicals.com/DIETHYLENE%20TRIAMINE %20PENTA%20ACETIC%20ACID%20MSDS%20LAB.htm.

4. "Should I Avoid Products with Triclosan?" *Mayo Clinic*. Accessed September 9, 2017, from http://www.mayoclinic.org/healthy-lifestyle/adult-health/ expert-answers/triclosan/faq-20057861.

5. "Trichloroisocyanuric acid." Accessed September 9, 2017, from https:// pubchem.ncbi.nlm.nih.gov/compound/Symclosene#section=Hazards-Identification.

PART IV

DETOX YOUR WARDROBE

1. *The True Cost*. Directed by Andrew Morgan. United States: Life Is My Movie Entertainment Company, 2015. https://truecostmovie.com/.

2. "Characteristics of Minimum Wage Workers, 2015." *Bureau of Labor Statistics*, United States Labor Department, April 2016. Accessed July 14, 2017, from https://www.bls.gov/opub/reports/minimum-wage/2015/home.htm.

CHAPTER 14

1. Nandita Raghuram, "Brands Are a Lot More Responsible for Terrible Factory Conditions Than They Want You to Think." *Racked*, May 2, 2017. Accessed July 14, 2017, from https://www.racked.com/2017/5/2/15425728/factory-conditions-brands-los-angeles-worker.

2. "Cotton: A Water Wasting Crop." *World Wildlife Fund*. Accessed July 14, 2017, from http://wwf.panda.org/about_our_earth/about_freshwater/freshwater_problems/thirsty_crops/cotton/.

3. "The Environmental Cost of Clothes." *China Water Risk*, April 18, 2011. Accessed July 14, 2017, from http://chinawaterrisk.org/resources/analysis-reviews/the-environmental-cost-of-clothes/.

4. Naga Munchetty, "Cambodia garment workers killed in clashes with police." *BBC News*, January 3, 2014. Accessed July 14, 2017, from http://www.bbc.com/news/av/world-asia-25585562/cambodia-garment-workers-killed-in-clashes-with-police.

5. OXFAM, "The Impact of the Second-Hand Clothing Trade on Developing Countries." Accessed September 10, 2017, from http://policy-practice.oxfam.org.uk/publications/the-impact-of-the-second-hand-clothing-trade-on-developing-countries-112464.

6. Gretchen Frazee, "How to stop 13 million tons of clothing from getting trashed every year." *PBS Newshour*, June 7, 2016. Accessed July 14, 2017, from http://www.pbs.org/newshour/updates/how-to-stop-13-million-tons-of-clothing-from-getting-trashed-every-year/.

7. Alden Wicker, "Fast Fashion Is Creating an Environmental Crisis." *Newsweek*, September 1, 2016. Accessed July 14, 2017, from http://www.newsweek.com/2016/09/09/old-clothes-fashion-waste-crisis-494824.html.

8. "About Us." Dutch Awearness company website. Accessed July 14, 2017, from http://dutchawearness.com/about/.

CHAPTER 15

1. "Death of a Child after Ingestion of a Metallic Charm—Minnesota, 2006." *Centers for Disease Control and Prevention*, last reviewed March 23, 2006. Accessed July 14, 2017, from https://www.cdc.gov/mmwr/preview/mmwrhtml/mm55d323a1.htm.

2. Adria Vasil, "Are plastic sandals leaching chemicals into my feet?" *Now Toronto*, July 7, 2011 Accessed July 14, 2017, from https://nowtoronto.com/lifestyle/ecoholic/are-plastic-sandals-leaching-chemicals-into-my-feet/.

3. http://nativeshoes.com/faq.

4. Elizabeth Grossman, "Are Flame Retardants Safe? Growing Evidence Says 'No.'" *Yale Environment 360* (New Haven, CT: Yale School of Forestry & Environmental Studies, September 29, 2011). Accessed July 14, 2017, from http://e360.yale.edu/features/pbdes_are_flame_retardants_safe_growing_evidence_says_no.

5. Clyde Haberman, "A Flame Retardant That Came with Its Own Threat to Health." *The New York Times*, May 3, 2015. Accessed July 14, 2017, from https://www.nytimes.com/2015/05/04/us/a-flame-retardant-that-came-with-its-own-threat-to-health.html?mcubz=1&_r=0.

6. Charlotte Cowles, "The Real Story on Organic Dry-Cleaning." *The New York Sun*, September 16, 2008. Accessed July 14, 2017, from http://www.nysun.com/style/the-real-story-on-organic-dry-cleaning/85914/.

7. Sian Anna Lewis, "The Dangers of Sheep Dip—the Essential Facts." *Country File Magazine*, July 1, 2015. Accessed July 14, 2017, from http://www.countryfile.com/explore-countryside/food-and-farming/dangers-sheep-dip-essential-facts.

8. Sally Gaw and Graham McBride, "Sheep Dip Factsheet: Sheep Dips in New Zealand." *Christchurch, New Zealand: Environment Southland*, December 2010. Accessed July 14, 2017, from http://www.es.govt.nz/Document%20Library/Factsheets/Pollution%20prevention%20factsheets/Sheep%20dip%20factsheets/sheep-dip-factsheet-1-sheep-dips-in-nz.pdf.

9. "Dipping." *New South Wales Government, Department of Primary Industries, Australia*. Accessed July 14, 2017, from http://www.dpi.nsw.gov.au/animals-and-livestock/animal-welfare/general/general-welfare-of-livestock/sop/sheep/health/dipping.

10. "Wool." *O Ecotextiles*, updated September 6, 2010. Accessed July 14, 2017, from https://oecotextiles.wordpress.com/category/fibers/wool/.

CHAPTER 16

1. "Breast cancer clusters: Why do some places have higher rates of breast cancer?" *Komen Perspectives*, Susan G. Komen website, October 24, 2011. Accessed

July 14, 2017, from http://ww5.komen.org/KomenPerspectives/Breast-cancer-clusters--why-do-some-places-have-higher-rates-of-breast-cancer-.html.

2. Michael Wyde, et al., "Report of Partial Findings from the National Toxicology Program Carcinogenesis Studies of Cell Phone Radiofrequency Radiation in Hsd: Sprague Dawley® SD rats (Whole Body Exposures)." *bioRxiv: The Preprint Server for Biology*, doi: https://doi.org/10.1101/055699, preprint first posted online May. 26, 2016. Accessed July 14, 2017, from http://www.biorxiv.org/content/biorxiv/early/2016/05/26/055699.full.pdf. As a note, his article is a preprint and has not been peer-reviewed.

3. Patrizia Frei, et al., "Use of mobile phones and risk of brain tumours: Update of Danish cohort study." *The BMJ*, 343 (2011): d6387, doi: https://doi.org/10.1136/bmj.d6387.

4. Fact Sheet No. 193, "Electromagnetic fields and public health: mobile phones." *World Health Organization*, reviewed October 2014. Accessed July 14, 2017, from http://www.who.int/mediacentre/factsheets/fs193/en/.

5. "Exposure and Testing Requirements for Mobile Phones Should Be Reassessed." *U.S. Government Accountability Office*, July 2012. Accessed July 14, 2017, from http://www.gao.gov/assets/600/592902.pdf.

6. Miller is also a FRCP, FRCP (C), FFPH, FACE, Professor Emeritus, Dalla Lana School of Public Health; Senior Medical Advisor, Environmental Health Trust, USA, and previous Director of Epidemiology, National Cancer Institute of Canada.

CHAPTER 17

1. William Pentland, "The Most Toxic Toys." *Forbes*, December 16, 2008. Accessed July 14, 2017, from https://www.forbes.com/2008/12/16/toys-product-safety-biz-commerce-cx_wp_1216toxictoys.html.

2. "Chemicals in Children's Toys: Addressing Stricter Limits and Environmental Concerns." *UL Environment White Paper*, 2012. Accessed July 14, 2017, from http://library.ul.com/wp-content/uploads/sites/40/2015/02/UL_WP_Final_Chemicals-in-Childrens-Toys_v5-HR.pdf.

3. Keely Chalmers, "Tests find toxic metals in children's Halloween makeup." *USA Today Network* (Portland, OR: KGW-TV, October 26, 2016). Accessed July 14, 2017, from https://www.usatoday.com/story/news/nation-now/2016/10/26toxic-metals-childrens-halloween-makeup/92759186/.

4. Deborah Kotz, "FDA warns against getting temporary tattoos." *Boston Globe*, April 1, 2013, Accessed July 14, 2017, from https://www.bostonglobe.com/lifestyle/health-wellness/2013/03/31/are-temporary-tattoos-toxic-fda-warns-against-them/fBILImVuLBd8e9Y3aLFAdN/story.html.

5. "How Toxic Materials in Toys Are Causing Children Health Problems?" *Bears for Humanity*, June 2003. Accessed July 14, 2017, from https://www

.bearsforhumanity.com/blogs/bear-blog/33548995-how-toxic-materials-in
-toys-are-causing-children-health-problems.

6. "Are Art Supplies Toxic?" *Green American Magazine*. Accessed July 14,
2017, from https://www.greenamerica.org/green-living/are-art-supplies-toxic.

7. Kathy, "SafeMama Play Dough Showdown," *SafeMama.com*, April 9,
2009. Accessed July 14, 2017, from http://safemama.com/2009/04/09
/safemama-play-dough-showdown/.

8. "3M™ LeadCheck™ Swabs Overview." *3M*. Accessed July 14, 2017,
from http://www.3m.com/3M/en_US/company-us/all-3m-products/~/All-3M
-Products/Consumer/Home-Improvement/3M-LeadCheck-Swabs/?N=50023
85+8709316+8740610+8743721+3294857497&rt=r3.

9. Jennifer Taylor, "Why Incredibly Dangerous Amber Teething Necklaces
Should Be Banned." *MomTricks*, July 12, 2017. accessed July 14, 2017, from
https://www.momtricks.com/babies/dangers-of-baltic-amber-teething
-necklaces/.

CHAPTER 18

1. Richard Stehouwer and Kirsten Macneal, "Lead in Residential Soils:
Sources, Testing, and Reducing Exposure." *Factsheet, Penn State College of Agricultural Sciences*, Pennsylvania State University: 2017. Accessed July 14, 2017,
from http://extension.psu.edu/plants/crops/esi/lead-in-soil.

2. Tony Barboza and Ben Poston, "Brain-damaging lead levels near battery
plant found as high as 100 times above health limits." *The Los Angeles Times*,
July 20, 2016. Accessed July 14, 2017, from http://www.latimes.com/local/
california/la-me-ln-dangerous-lead-levels-20160714-snap-story.html.

3. Clyde Haberman, "A Flame Retardant That Came with Its Own Threat
to Health." *The New York Times*, May 3, 2015. Accessed July 14, 2017, from
https://www.nytimes.com/2015/05/04/us/a-flame-retardant-that-came-with
-its-own-threat-to-health.html?mcubz=1&_r=0.

4. Jane Sheppard, "Prevent Toxic Off-Gassing When You Can't Afford
to Buy an Organic Mattress." *Healthy Child*, November 5, 2013. Accessed
July 14, 2017, from https://www.healthychild.com/prevent-toxic-off-gassing
-when-you-cant-afford-to-buy-an-organic-mattress/.

5. Cambria Bold, "Healthy Sleep Pillows: 6 All-Natural and Non-Toxic
Options." *Apartment Therapy*, August 16, 2011. Accessed July 14, 2017, from
http://www.apartmenttherapy.com/healthy-pillows-6-natural-nont-136344.

6. "Ten Myths of Lead Paint." *Occupational Knowledge International*. Accessed
July 14, 2017, from http://www.okinternational.org/lead-paint/Myths.

7. Rebecca Kessler, "Lead-Based Decorative Paints: Where Are They Still
Sold—and Why?" *Environmental Health Perspectives*, 122(4), (April 2014):
A96–A103. doi: 10.1289/ehp.122-A96.

8. "Renovation, Repair, and Painting (RRP) Rule: Frequent Questions." *U.S. Environmental Protection Agency*, August 11, 2014. Accessed July 14, 2017, from https://www.epa.gov/sites/production/files/2014-09/documents/full_rrp_fqs_-august_11_2014.pdf.

9. "Garden Hose Study." *Ann Arbor, MI: Ecology Center*, June 2016. Accessed July 14, 2017, from http://ecocenter.org/sites/default/files/healthy-stuff/images/Garden%20Hose%20Report%20June%2020%202016.pdf.

INDEX

ABOUT THE AUTHOR

Christine Dimmick is a health and wellness advocate, activist, and founder of the Good Home Company, Inc. (www.goodhome.com). Christine was one of the first pioneers to create natural cleaning products more than twenty years ago in her New York City kitchen. She spreads awareness on the toxins in our life with regular speaking engagements at Canyon Ranch Lenox, JCC NYC, and in local communities where it is needed most. Christine actively works with non-profits, nongovernmental organizations, startups, and organizations helping to create new solutions for the future of water, farming, and our environment. With the creation of conscious gatherings (community gatherings in health and wellness), Christine hopes to empower people with the facts and sources so they can make more sustainable and healthy choices. She and Good Home products have been featured in *Real Simple*, *O Magazine*, *InStyle*, *Dr. Oz*, along with appearances on the *Today* show. Christine lives in New York City's historic Seaport district with her husband, son, and rescue Chihuahua, Ringo. To reach Christine, visit www.christinedimmick.com.